Lifestyle Redesign
Implementing the Well Elderly Program

DATE DUE

Deborah R. Mandel, MA, OTR
Jeanne M. Jackson, PhD, OTR
Ruth Zemke, PhD, OTR, FAOTA
Laurie Nelson, MA, OTR
Florence A. Clark, PhD, OTR, FAOTA

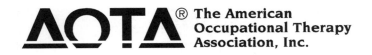
AOTA® The American Occupational Therapy Association, Inc.

The American Occupational Therapy Association, Inc.
4720 Montgomery Lane
PO Box 31220
Bethesda, Maryland 20824-1220

Disclaimers
This publication is designed to provide accurate and authoritative information in regard to the subject matter covered. It is sold or distributed with the understanding that the publisher is not engaged in rendering legal, accounting, or other professional service. If legal advice or other expert assistance is required, the services of a competent professional person should be sought.
  From the Declaration of Principles jointly adopted by the American Bar Association
  and a Committee of Publishers and Associations

It is the objective of The American Occupational Therapy Association to be a forum for free expression and interchange of ideas. The opinions expressed by the contributors to this work are their own and not necessarily those of either the editors or The American Occupational Therapy Association.

ISBN 1-56900-120-0

Dedication

To all of the participants in the USC Well Elderly Program

Contents

Acknowledgments

We thank the four occupational therapists—Laura Caron-Parker, Shan-Pin Fanchiang, Pei-Fen Chang, and Laurie Nelson, who implemented the University of Southern California (USC) Well Elderly Program and shared their expertise and creativity. We likewise acknowledge the contributions of other members of the USC Well Elderly Study team: Michael Carlson, Stanley P. Azen, Loren G. Lipson, Joel W. Hay, Barbara Cherry, and Karen Josephson. Without their efforts, there would be no *Lifestyle Redesign* manual.

The USC Well Elderly Study was funded by the National Institute on Aging; the National Center for Medical Rehabilitation Research; the Agency for Health Care Policy and Research; the American Occupational Therapy Foundation Center at USC for the Study of Occupation and Its Relations to Adaptation; the RGK Foundation; Lumex, Inc.; and Smith and Nephew Roylan.

About the Authors

Deborah R. Mandel, MA, OTR, is an instructor of clinical occupational therapy and a doctoral student at the University of Southern California (USC). She was the project coordinator for the Well Elderly Study funded by the National Institute on Aging and the American Occupational Therapy Foundation.

Jeanne M. Jackson, PhD, OTR, is an assistant professor at USC and was a co-investigator in the Well Elderly Study. Her research focuses on the symbolic aspects of occupation, especially how individuals create authentic lives through engaging in occupations.

Ruth Zemke, PhD, OTR, FAOTA, is a professor and graduate programs coordinator at USC. She was co-principal investigator for the Well Elderly Study and is an internationally recognized leader in the application of theories of occupation to clinical practice.

Laurie Nelson, MA, OTR, is a project specialist for the Well Elderly Study at USC. She was one of the four therapists who implemented the preventative occupational treatment for the seniors who participated in the Well Elderly Study.

Florence A. Clark, PhD, OTR, FAOTA, is professor and chair of the Department of Occupational Science and Occupational Therapy at USC. She was principal investigator for the Well Elderly Study and is a widely published and noted scholar in the field of occupational therapy.

Introduction

Before, I thought to retire meant waiting to die. Now I don't think so!
I'd like to work if I can; I want to learn.

Andrew Chu, Well Elderly Group participant, 1994

The University of Southern California (USC) Well Elderly Study determined that preventive occupational therapy greatly enhances the health and quality of life of independent-living older adults. This landmark study reaffirmed foundational principles in the fields of occupational science and occupational therapy. The USC Well Elderly Study was successful because of its focus on the core concept of occupation, which is not a new concept. Rather, the concept has been central to occupational therapy since the profession's establishment at the beginning of the 20th century. The principle of occupation-centered practice, combined with others, was cultivated and used to create a process called *occupational lifestyle redesign*. "Occupational lifestyle redesign is the process of developing and enacting a customized routine of health promoting and meaningful daily activities" (F. A. Clark, personal communication, July 8, 1998).

This manual provides a conceptual yet practical framework that enables occupational therapy practitioners to integrate the program's concepts into daily practice. The ideas and examples presented are not only relevant for elderly persons living independently, but also they can be applied in numerous settings with other populations to enhance individual treatment as well as group process. This manual is pertinent to all occupational therapists who are concerned with quality care and intervention at the earliest opportunity and who emphasize prevention of illness. Additionally, the content is useful for practitioners who are interested in helping their clients achieve more satisfying and meaningful lifestyles after catastrophic illness and disability.

The originators of the USC Well Elderly Study hope that this manual will increase awareness and recognition of skills you are already using in practice. The manual provides the terminology and framework for successful occupational therapy intervention with a focus on lifestyle redesign. It outlines the steps for a program that encourages incorporating your own self-reflection as a health care provider. As an occupational therapist, you have the education, training, and mindset to carry out the well-grounded concepts summarized in this manual.

As we experience the current financial struggles in health care, the profession of occupational therapy must market its resources and identify major outcomes for services. The USC Well Elderly Study provided compelling data that demonstrate the health benefits of preventive intervention. Preventive occupation-centered therapy improves elderly health-related quality of life (Clark et al., 1997) and reduces health-related costs.

This manual will bring greater importance to your group facilitation and individualized interventions. It will refine your understanding of occupational storytelling, occupational storymaking, and occupational self-analysis and assist you in showing clients how to walk through this process. This manual will support you in creating a lifestyle redesign program and in making evaluations and adaptations as necessary to maintain an individualized treatment focus.

We anticipate that all occupational therapists will be able to use the concepts of occupational lifestyle redesign in their daily practice. We encourage and challenge you to seek out potential adaptations in the areas where you practice. Make a difference! Our goal is to affirm the importance of occupation-centered practice, allow for a greater understanding of the concepts behind your methods, and make occupational therapy more meaningful to you and the clients whose lives you touch.

Deborah R. Mandel, MA, OTR
Jeanne M. Jackson, PhD, OTR
Ruth Zemke, PhD, OTR, FAOTA
Laurie Nelson, MA, OTR
Florence A. Clark, PhD, OTR, FAOTA

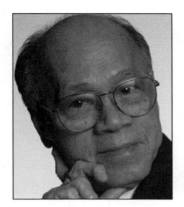

1

The USC Well Elderly Clinical Trial

The participants who were randomly assigned to the occupational therapy intervention in the University of Southern California (USC) (Los Angeles, CA) Well Elderly Study engaged in lifestyle redesign for 9 months. One of the most exciting elements of this process was that the participants in this group, on average, either maintained or improved their health-related quality of life and life satisfaction (Figure 1). Furthermore, the study was designed in such a way that it is clear that these changes were the result of a program of occupation-centered therapy and not merely involvement in activity. This occupational therapy program was therapeutic in that it provided independent-living elderly persons with the tools to analyze their own occupations, which enabled them to understand and alter their approaches to everyday activities, thereby optimizing function and well-being. The process was accomplished over time through experience, trial and error, risk taking, and coaching by an occupational therapist.

The second encouraging aspect of the USC Well Elderly Study was that it scientifically demonstrated that working with persons at the level of meaningful occupations is effective. In clinical settings, it is difficult to document occupational changes, and this leads to measuring the outcomes or results of occupational therapy techniques or components of occupation, which are

admittedly only a part of what occupational therapists do. Later in this chapter, we present the results of the USC Well Elderly Study in more detail.

The roots of the Lifestyle Redesign Program reach back into the rich soil of a century of occupational therapy practice, as well as the fertile fields of occupational science. We hope that an understanding of the design of the USC Well Elderly Study and its results will provide a foundation to empower your practice and enrich how you view and talk about occupational therapy to other practitioners, clients, professionals, and students. In the section that follows, we describe the series of studies and projects that contribute to the design effectiveness of the Lifestyle Redesign Program.

Constructing the Lifestyle Redesign Program

Figure 2 depicts the complex process of constructing the occupational therapy treatment protocol used in the USC Well Elderly Study, which became what we now call the Lifestyle Redesign Program. Various conceptual paths that arose from many directions led to the development of the USC Well Elderly Study. These included pilot studies, a demonstration class, and theoretical readings.

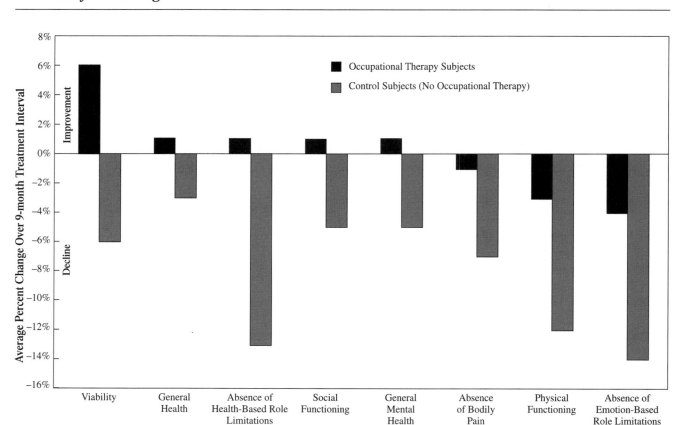

Figure 1. Well Elderly Study results: occupational therapy improves health and slows aging-related declines.

By presenting the historical progression that led up to the study, we hope that readers will fully understand the complexity of the project.

A pilot study and a demonstration class provided a broad understanding of aging, adaptation, and the process of occupational self-analysis. Two additional studies contributed more focused information on the local situation of the elderly persons whom we knew would be USC Well Elderly Study participants. These two studies were conducted with the prospect of the USC Well Elderly Study in mind. In turn, the resulting USC Well Elderly Study protocol provided the framework for the Lifestyle Redesign Program. Each of these preliminary steps is discussed in greater detail.

Living a Meaningful Existence in Old Age

The first pilot study was a qualitative study titled "Living a Meaningful Existence in Old Age" (Jackson, 1996), which was completed in 1992 during the time that the principal investigator was first considering a large study

of elderly persons and their occupations. The purpose of this pilot study was to identify adaptive strategies used by community-dwelling elderly persons with disabilities. The author followed a group of "exemplars," or elderly persons who were living successfully in the community. The findings revealed that sustaining symbolically meaningful lives entailed

- engaging in occupations saturated with themes of meaning,
- exercising control in the selection of occupations,
- seizing opportunities to take risks,
- modifying the environment to enhance accessibility to occupations,
- maintaining social connectedness, and
- sustaining an occupational temporal rhythm.

"Living a Meaningful Existence in Old Age" (Jackson, 1996) became an umbrella study that turned our attention to some broad issues in aging and adaptation. For example, we paid particular attention to the ways in which these elderly respondents sought risks and to the kinds of activities they would experience as risky. For example, for one respondent, speaking at a Toastmasters club was perceived as a considerable risk. This quest for challenge was not necessarily desired on a daily basis, but rather every now and then, tucked away in the overall pattern of occupation. Simply stated, the respondent craved intermittent or occasional excitement.

At this time, we began to define our conceptualization of themes of meaning. We noticed how the elderly persons interpreted their present daily occupations in terms of their overarching themes of meaning. Additionally, the pilot study raised questions in our minds about the nature of occupation itself. For example, we wondered about the distinction between *imagining* and *doing*. One respondent, Ruth, was sequestered to a chair in her mobile home due to her orthopedic limitations yet claimed that she experienced vicarious pleasure by reliving gardening in her mind. By evoking sentiments, visual imagery, and the physical sensibilities (Jackson, 1996) associated with this previous occupation, she was able to venture mentally into her garden and plant. Would we call this kind of preoccupation an "occupation?"

Occupational Self-Analysis

The second step was the development of a process called *occupational self-analysis*, which Clark conceptualized during a class she taught at USC. During this course, students successfully analyzed their own occupational patterns and modified their lifestyles to maximize productivity and life satisfaction. They reflected on who they are as occupational beings, how their childhood occupations shaped their adult characters, and how the things they do each day contribute to or compromise their health and well-being. Hundreds of students took the class and underwent this self-reflection process. They learned to focus their attention on how they select occupations each day and whether their everyday routines were a sensible plan for achieving goals. The class became incredibly popular and grew in enrollment during the years Dr. Clark taught it. The enthusiasm of the students for occupational self-analysis suggested that this might be an effective approach for other populations, such as elderly persons.

Adaptive Strategies

Although the previously described initial study and class provided clues for a broad conceptualization of the occu-

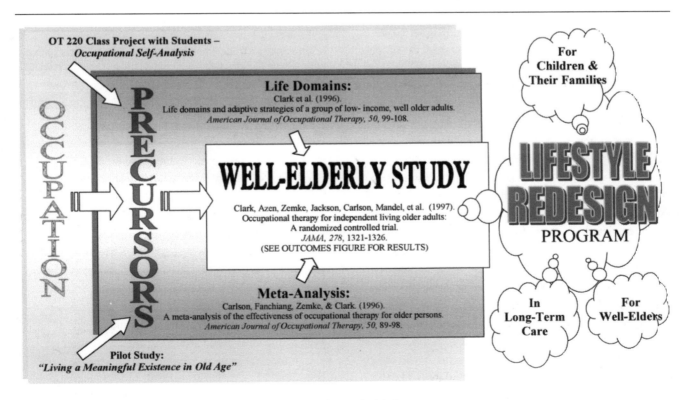

Figure 2. The emergence of the Lifestyle Redesign Program for Well Elderly participants.

pational treatment that would be used in the USC Well Elderly Study, we realized that the protocol would need to be sensitive to the local situations of the participants. Consequently, we conducted a pilot study to uncover knowledge about the concerns of the persons targeted for the large effectiveness study. Ten domains emerged from the data as areas of key concern to this group (i.e., areas in which they perceived they needed help):

1. Activities of daily living (ADL)
2. Adaptation to a multicultural environments
3. Use of free time
4. Grave illness and death
5. Health maintenance
6. Health mobility
7. Personal finances
8. Personal safety
9. Psychological well-being and happiness
10. Relationships with others

The importance of this study was that, although some of these domains (i.e., personal safety, ADL) are typically included in occupational therapy, other domains were not anticipated. For example, adaptation to a multicultural environment is not typically included in a formalized or focused way in occupational therapy. Unfortunately, in this particular setting, various elderly persons were having problems coexisting with persons of different ethnicities. Having once lived in ethnically isolated neighborhoods, they now found themselves in a huge apartment complex centrally located in downtown Los Angeles where persons of various ethnicities are housed together. Problems, as well as prejudicial attitudes, surfaced and were embedded in daily occupations.

For example, using the elevator (which was essential in this high-rise setting) became a catalyst in aggravating stereotypes about neighbors from different cultures. Those elderly persons from cultures that put a premium on time were more likely to approach the elevator, push the button, enter, and go. However, elderly persons from cultures that put greater value on community would often hold the elevator door open for a substantial amount of time either to have a conversation or to allow a friend who was halfway down the hall to enter the elevator. Again, the study highlighted the importance of customizing a program to the local situation because this domain (adaptation to a multicultural environment) would not be relevant with a more homogeneous population. For this reason, we recommend that practitioners conduct a

detailed needs evaluation of the elderly persons with whom they will be implementing the Lifestyle Redesign Program and modify the modules accordingly.

Meta-Analysis

Finally, a meta-analysis of the effectiveness of occupational therapy for older persons was conducted (Carlson, Fanchiang, Zemke, & Clark, 1996). Meta-analysis is a statistical procedure that can give information about the likelihood of treatment success, or lack of success, on the basis of the combined findings of similar research studies. The results of this study indicated "a highly significant cumulative result for treatment success ($p < 0.001$)" (Carlson et al., 1996, p. 89), which suggested that an outcome study on the effectiveness of occupational therapy with elderly persons, provided it had sufficient power, was likely to yield positive findings. One important result of this meta-analysis was that it gave us confidence to forge ahead with the USC Well Elderly Study.

Conclusion

In summary, the design of the USC Well Elderly Study, and particularly that of the occupational therapy protocol (now called the Lifestyle Redesign Program), was constructed through the implementation of several pilot studies. These studies provided insight into the more general as well as the local concerns of the elderly persons who would participate in the USC Well Elderly Study. In addition, the principal investigator's experience in developing a process of occupational self-analysis and its success over time informed the design of the Lifestyle Redesign Program. Implementation of the program in other settings would not require the same time- and resource-consuming process we have described. Instead, we recommend that practitioners use the Lifestyle Redesign Program as a template that should be modified by the findings of a local needs evaluation.

A needs evaluation at each site allows the practitioner to elicit the factors associated with life satisfaction, health, and productivity that are idiosyncratic to each group of elderly persons. We recommend that, in thinking about modifying the Lifestyle Redesign Program, practitioners read articles that we have cited in each chapter for background information and to inform fully the modification process for their local situation.

In the next section, we describe the results of the USC Well Elderly Study in detail. In implementing the Lifestyle Redesign Program, occupational therapists must be advocates for the efficiency and cost effectiveness of the program. The following section provides model ways to be successful in this role.

Talking About the Results

The early studies delineated in the previous section trace the roots of the USC Well Elderly Study. The meta-analysis examined a body of occupational therapy interventions with elderly persons, and this work substantiated that occupational therapy can be effective with this population. This study had two results. First, it became apparent that a single, large study was needed that would test the effectiveness of occupational therapy. Second, the study gave the Well Elderly team the confidence to attempt a larger study. The implication of the meta-analysis was that it would be possible to demonstrate a positive benefit of occupational therapy, provided that we could construct a sufficiently rigorous research design that would be sensitive to detecting changes due to the occupational therapy intervention (Box 1). The results of the USC Well Elderly Study indicated that this was correct, and the study was published as the lead article in the *Journal of the American Medical Association* (*JAMA*) on October 22, 1997 (Clark et al., 1997). The principle investigator, Florence A. Clark, was invited to address the American Medical Association 16th Annual Science Reporters Conference on October 21, 1997, to present the results. Her speech is included here to give the reader a model language through which to convey the findings of the USC Well Elderly Study and the potential effect of the Lifestyle Redesign Program on elderly persons and the health care system.

Remarks by Dr. Clark

"I'm here to talk to you about the Well Elderly Study, the largest study ever conducted in the field of occupational therapy. It was recently completed at the University of Southern California with funding from the National Institutes of Health and the American Occupational Therapy Foundation, and it indicates that preventive occupational therapy can have a tremendous impact on the elderly by improving physical and mental health, increasing vitality, and slowing declines in physical functioning, bodily pain, and emotion-based limitations.

"These findings are exciting because they demonstrate occupational therapy as an effective way to promote health and increase quality of life for America's

rapidly growing elderly population. Our research results show promise for helping senior citizens maintain their independence. This is crucial because it is the loss of independence that strikes fear in the hearts of many elderly people—and it is the high cost of dependent care

Box 1
The Advantages of Randomization

The USC Well Elderly Study was a randomized clinical trial. All participants were assigned randomly to one of three groups after they completed a battery of questionnaires and were screened by a geriatrician. The three groups were (a) occupational therapy (lifestyle redesign), (b) social activity control, and (c) no treatment control.

The process of randomization is one of the most important reasons that the results of the USC Well Elderly Study are reliable. In any research with humans, especially research conducted in the "real world," it is difficult to know if any change is actually a result of the intervention. There are myriad reasons unrelated to the intervention that cause one person to change for the better and another to change for the worse. The outcome of the person whose health indices decline may have been affected by an undiagnosed illness, worry about a sick grandchild, or a decline in the stock market.

When research participants are randomized and the sample size is large enough, it is highly likely that persons who have conditions in their lives that might negatively affect the results of an intervention have been evenly distributed among the three groups. Consequently, these effects can be ignored when comparing the groups because they are equally distributed. This is likewise true for positive effects. The benefit from an intervention may be greater for someone with a particular type of personality or a certain level of education. Randomization ensures that these positive effects will be evenly distributed across the three groups. With randomization, it is not necessary to identify any of the factors (including those not even imagined) that might influence the effectiveness of an intervention. Because of the process of randomization, it is accepted that any differences in outcome measures that arise when the groups are compared must be due to the intervention.

that threatens the financial security of millions of Americans as well as the health care system that serves us all.

"Before discussing the USC Well Elderly Study in more detail, I want to take a moment to define *occupational therapy* for you. As a health profession, occupational therapy focuses on the goal of helping people experience healthy and satisfying lives by maximizing their ability to successfully accomplish everyday activities—activities that we term occupations. It's not physical therapy, although there's a physical element involved. It's not psychotherapy, although there's a psychological element involved. While counseling can be thought of as a *talking* therapy, occupational therapy is a *doing* therapy.

"Occupational therapists draw upon their expertise in anatomy, physiology, psychology, anthropology, sociology, and human development to prescribe for their clients a customized plan of occupations that will promote their well-being. Just as there is no one diet that meets the health needs of every American, there is no one prescription of activities that guarantees optimum health and happiness for everyone. What occupational therapists do is customized lifestyle redesign.

"Occupational therapists have traditionally worked with populations that face special challenges, such as the sick or those with a disability. But they can help all individuals understand and redesign their lifestyles to be happier, more productive, independent members of society. Simply put, physicians can help people live longer, while occupational therapists can show people how to live better.

"There is another term you should know about—one you will hear more of in the future, and that's *occupational science*. It is an academic discipline that focuses on the critical role of daily activities in promoting health and a sense of well-being in our lives on the nature of occupation and its effects on human beings. Sometimes, occupational scientists mine the traditional social sciences such as anthropology, psychology, and sociology to extract knowledge specifically focused on the impact of meaningful activity or occupations on health, self-image, and productivity. Occupational science examines questions such as

- What are the contributions of work and leisure to physical health, happiness, and quality of life?
- What is the relationship between childhood occupations and adult competency and achievement?

- What constitutes a healthy balance of work, rest, and leisure on a typical day?

"Occupational scientists, occupational therapists, and physicians at USC conducted the Well Elderly Study, a large-scale experiment designed to assess whether preventive occupational therapy does in fact lead to improved health and well-being in older adults. The research subjects were 361 seniors, age 60 to 89, who were drawn from federally subsidized apartment buildings for low-income older adults in greater Los Angeles. These men and women were quite culturally diverse and included African-Americans, Hispanics, whites, and Asians. In fact, to meet the needs of this population, we conducted all our activities in both Mandarin and English (Box 2). And because our sample was so diverse, we believe our results are applicable across the country and across all ethnic groups.

"Our study subjects were randomly divided into 3 groups. One group received professionally led occupational therapy, another group participated in social activities coordinated by nonprofessionals, and a third group received no programs at all. The seniors in the occupational therapy group participated in weekly 2-hr group sessions conducted by a registered occupational therapist and also received another hour a month of individual occupational therapy. The fact that the majority of the occupational therapy was conducted in group sessions is a cost-effective method of providing services, which means OT (occupational therapy) can be efficiently delivered on a widespread basis to large numbers of people.

Box 2
Who Were the
USC Well Elderly Study Participants?

Senior citizens (60 years of age and older)

- Low income
- Living independently
- Urban
- Multiethnic
- 30% Mandarin Chinese speakers
- 70% English speakers
- 65% Women
- 73% Lived alone
- 27% With disabilities (as defined by the participant)

"The social activity control group participated in weekly sessions lasting 2 1/4 hr, during which time a coordinator without professional training conducted activities such as community outings, dances, games, movies, and craft projects.

"All participants were evaluated at the beginning of the study and 9 months later—at the end (Figure 3)—with tests that measured physical health, social functioning, mental health, and life satisfaction (Box 3). The fact that our study extended over such a relatively long period of time—9 months—enhances the significance of the findings, as does our use of the RAND 36-Item Health Status Survey (SF-36; Hays, Sherbourne, & Mazel, 1993; Ware & Sherbourne, 1992), widely regarded as the 'gold standard' measure for assessing a person's physical and psychological health status.

"Our findings show that the subjects who received occupational therapy experienced more positive gains and fewer declines than did the subjects in the two control groups. In particular, the seniors who received occupational therapy showed improvement in 5 of the 8 SF-36 general categories measured, while the control groups recorded declines across the board. Some of the results were notable. In the area of limitation in work and activities due to physical health problems, the OT group showed an increase of 1%, while the control groups declined by 13%, for a 14% difference. In the measure of vitality, the OT group showed an increase of 6%, while the control groups declined by 2%, for an 8% difference. Other areas of improvement in the OT group showed differences of 4 to 6% better than the control group.

"Even in the three areas where occupational therapy was not able to improve the health level of the elderly participants, the OT group showed significantly less deterioration than the control groups. For example, in the area of limitations in work and activities due to emotional problems, the OT group declined by 4%, whereas the control groups declined by 14%, for a 10% difference. In the area of physical functioning, the OT group declined by 3%, while the non–occupational therapy groups declined by 12%, producing a 9% difference.

"What did the occupational therapists do to make this happen? The occupational therapists attempted to

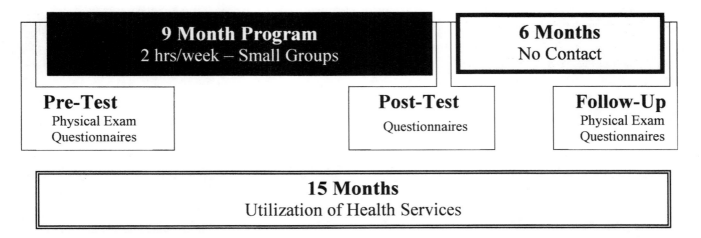

Figure 3. Timeline for the Well Elderly Study.

help participants better understand and appreciate the importance of meaningful activity in their lives, as well as teach them how to select and perform activities so they could achieve a healthy and satisfying lifestyle. Subjects learned how to alter their approach to everyday activities such as shopping, grooming, exercising, and doing hobbies in order to maximize function, vitality, and productivity. The therapy included both instruction and safety, public transportation, nutrition, exercise, and energy conservation. Therapists worked with clients to assess the amount of activity they were engaged in; the meaningfulness of these activities; their beliefs, values, attitudes and goals; and balance within their daily routines. The process resulted in the development of a comprehensive individualized plan designed to promote a healthier and more meaningful life.

"For example, an 80-year-old woman who was depressed spent most of her days in bed or watching television. She rarely ventured out of her building because she was unfamiliar with public transportation and was afraid of falling when taking that first 'big step' to climb aboard a bus. The occupational therapist created a step in her apartment that matched the height of the step up from the street to the bus and then assisted her client in practicing that skill. Once the woman possessed sufficient confidence, the therapist escorted her on a trip by bus and then coached her to make several trips out on her own. The bus step then became a symbolic threshold to a whole world of new experiences with radiating health benefits. The woman later reported that these experiences gave her a new lease on life and that she felt healthier than she had in many years.

"Many of the elderly men and women in our OT group reported similar experiences and benefits. In contrast, neither the social activity group nor the non-activity group experienced any improvement in health or well-being. And in all measures where decline was documented across the study group, occupational therapy was shown to substantially slow this decline.

"What are the ramifications of the USC Well Elderly Study? First, our research demonstrates that a preventive occupational therapy program can help seniors remain healthy and independent for a greater period of time. This is likely, over the long run, to keep them out of hospitals and nursing homes. The end result is that they can experience healthier, happier lives.

"Second, because healthy and independent is less expensive than sick and dependent, our study sends an

important message to the health care industry. We may be able to reduce morbidity and the effects of disability—and at the same time reduce costs—by adopting occupational therapy as a preventive tool in our health care arsenal. The government currently spends $45 billion, or approximately 60%, of its Medicare and Medicaid budget on nursing home care. Ultimately, it may be in everyone's interest for managed care and government health programs to include coverage of preventive occupational therapy in their plans.

"Third, our findings argue against the cliché that 'Keeping busy keeps you healthy.' We found that the elderly men and women who were regularly involved in social activity fared no better or worse than those who did not receive any treatment at all. This suggests that professional direction is a necessary ingredient in producing the therapeutic effects that can result from engagement in activity.

"Finally, the positive results of the USC Well Elderly Study demonstrate the applicability of occupational therapy practice to a new frontier—the preventive arena. What we do everyday, and how we do it over our lifetime, has a cumulative effect on our health. Eventually, it may determine whether we can live alone in older age or have to enter a nursing home. A critical key to independence is having a history of health-promoting occupation.

"In addition to assisting individuals who already have illness or disability, occupational therapists can apply their skills to helping people who have not yet had a catastrophe—people who can learn and practice the skills to lead longer, happier, and more satisfying lives."

It should be noted that *JAMA* reported the results of comparing preintervention testing with that completed immediately after the 9-month intervention (Clark et al., 1997). The participants were evaluated 6 months after the end of the intervention (see Box 1). Participants were additionally surveyed throughout the 15-month study period for their use of health care resources. The latter made it possible to analyze whether the Lifestyle Redesign Program is cost effective as well as beneficial for health and well-being. The results of these analyses, which to date have not yet been published, indicate that the effects of the occupational therapy intervention were sustained after 6 months and that this intervention is a cost-effective health strategy.

In chapter 2, we will delve more deeply into the conceptual foundation of the Lifestyle Redesign Program. The historical roots of how occupation has been understood in occupational therapy will be traced, and we will discuss how the focus on occupation is emphasized in the Lifestyle Redesign Program. Key concepts from occupational science that have informed the derivation of the Lifestyle Redesign Program will likewise be addressed.   ■

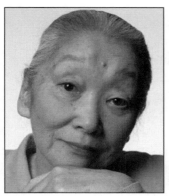

2
Lifestyle Redesign Program: Conceptual Foundation

Occupation, the core concept of occupational therapy, has a rich history that began with the founders of the National Society for the Promotion of Occupation Therapy, which was later renamed the American Occupational Therapy Association. The founders' descriptions of the curative effect of occupations laid the foundation for a truly unique profession—occupational therapy.

Peloquin (1991a) proposed a framework for understanding the continuity of occupation as a concept that is extended through time. Specifically, she stated that occupation is "a seminal idea [that] can be extended while also being shaped in time" (p. 353). As Peloquin suggested, the perception of occupation and its use as a therapeutic tool has taken various forms throughout our history.

Early in the profession, productive or meaningful occupation was the core of occupational therapy in the sense that, when customized to the patient, occupation was viewed as health promoting and essential to living a quality life. The goal of occupational therapy was to enable persons to be involved in meaningful, productive, and satisfying occupation because of the positive effect of occupation on health. Occupational therapy practitioners were lifestyle redesigners.

However, as some historians and scholars have argued, occupational therapy eventually went through a period in which the focus of therapy was on the components or substrates of occupation. For example, Reed (1986) described the situation in which a patient is set up to use a bilateral sander for strengthening the shoulder but given no sandpaper or purpose in mind. In fact, this activity does have a purpose (strengthening muscle) that may contribute to laying a foundation for better functional performance in the future and, therefore, a more engaged life. What distinguishes this example from the theories of the founders, however, is the degree of focus on a substrate of occupation rather than on the person as an occupational being, a person who needs a customized plan of daily occupation that will be health promoting.

Current health care policies present their own social challenges and opportunities. On one hand, "function" has become the primary justification for insurance reimbursement. Thus, occupational therapy practitioners, who benefit from 90 years of expertise in assisting persons to live meaningful lives through their ability to function, are in the forefront of health care. On the other hand, cutbacks in time spent with patients—mandated by health care—stifles treatment possibilities. The Lifestyle Redesign Program is one answer to these challenges in health care. Grounded solidly in occupation, the protocol reaches back in history to the roots of occupational therapy and offers an occupation-based treatment that is viable in contemporary times.

Our intent is to demonstrate how the Lifestyle Redesign Program is both grounded in the early founders' ideologies and is an extension of their ideals shaped by time, social conditions, and cultural ideologies. To a certain extent, the Lifestyle Redesign Program is not a new concept but rather is a refined contemporary version of what occupational therapy practitioners have traditionally done and is accessible to all practitioners through its core properties.

Core Ideas of the Lifestyle Redesign Program

In the following section, we list core ideas of the Lifestyle Redesign Program and illustrate how they have always been central to the beliefs of occupational therapy leaders.

1. Occupational therapy practitioners have long honored the essential necessity of occupation for human existence. In fact, the unique feature of the profession is its belief that active participation in occupation is life itself.

Early on, as well as in recent years, the all-important connection between occupation and life satisfaction has been the foundation of the profession. Dunton (as cited in Peloquin, 1991b) stated that "occupation is as necessary to life as food and drink" (p. 734). In 1920, Barton claimed that a human "is not a normal man just because his temperature is 98.6. A man is not a normal man until he is able to provide for himself" (as cited in Peloquin, 1991a, p. 355). He believed that to "merely get the patient well is not the whole thing, but to get him well for something" (p. 355). For Barton, that something was proper occupation providing "the basis or a corollary of a new life upon recovery" (p. 355). Meyer (1977) suggested that

> Our body is not merely so many pounds of flesh and bone figuring as a machine, with an abstract mind or soul added to it. It is throughout a live organism, pulsating with its rhythm of rest and activity, beating time (as we might say) in ever so many ways most readily intelligible, and in the full bloom of its nature when it feels itself as one of those great self-guiding energy-transformers which constitute the real world of living beings. Our conception of man is that of an organism that maintains and balances itself in the world of reality and actuality by being in active life and active use, i.e. using and living and acting its time in harmony with its own nature and the nature about it. It is the use that we make of ourselves that gives ultimate stamp to our every organ. (p. 641)

Jane Addams (1990), a cofounder of Hull House, which had a major influence on occupational therapy, drew on Huxley's work and stated that "the sense of uselessness is the severest shock which the human system can sustain, and that if persistently sustained, it results in atrophy of function" (p. 71). Yerxa et al. (1989) stated that "Individuals are most true to their humanity when engaged in occupation" (p. 7).

2. In affirming the occupational nature of humans, leaders in the profession have conceptualized the ways in which the experience of occupation creates a vision of new possible selves and life changes.

Occupational therapy scholars have always acknowledged the patient's ability to create occupational scenes where they envision themselves absorbed in meaningful occupations. Fazio (1992) stated that occupational therapy helps people "to see things differently, to present them with options, and to help them feel differently about the things they see" (p. 118). Tracy (as cited in Peloquin, 1991a) emphasized this purpose of occupations, stating that "If a nurse can prove to the patient who chafes against his limitations that there is really a broad highway of usefulness opening before him of which he knows not, the mental friction is diminished and satisfaction steals in" (p. 356). Occupations have the power of inducing patients' visions of a future life worth living because, through participation in occupations, they begin to comprehend the possibilities available to them. As one patient of occupational therapy commented in 1918, "I got a new vision of life . . ." (Cooper, as cited in Peloquin, 1991b, p. 735).

3. In thinking about the function of occupation, leaders in the field have addressed its effect on physical and mental health and on life order and routine.

The inherent value of occupation to promote health is a key belief in the profession, although it has taken on different nuances of meaning with changing times. A few quotes from leaders in the field of occupational therapy provide a sense of both continuity and change throughout the years. Dunton (1915), reading a hospital annual report stated,

> The amusements provided in the establishment for lunatics, as draughts, chess, backgammon, nine pins, swinging, sawing wood, gardening, reading, writing music etc . . . afford exercise both of body and mind [and] have a powerful effect in tranquilizing the mind, breaking up wrong associations of ideas and inducing correct habits of thinking as well as acting. (p. 12)

Hall (1918) stated,

> The cement flowerpot workers gave me an actual thrill. Here was a group of people who would ordinarily be degenerating in idleness. They were not only gaining self confidence and efficiency, they were actually adding to the world's supply of usable commodities, they were earning a little money which would help to keep them self-respecting. (p. 38)

Tracy (1912) commented,

> When the work is followed for its own sake, wholesome interests are substituted for morbid ones and gradually the attention is shifted to and absorbed by the new lines of thought aroused, so that, instead of being a medicine that can be dropped when the patient is cured, it has become rather a part of the restored individual's life, to be retained in some form so long as health exists. Such a result means a cure in the broadest sense, in that the mental attitude toward life has been changed. Wholesome interests have been aroused, and a conscious poise and control in the use of one's strength in the accomplishment of work has made work a pleasure and life satisfying. (pp. 2–3)

Slagle (1921) wrote that "Occupations used remedially serve to overcome some habits, to modify others and construct new ones, to the end that habit reactions will be favorable to the restoration and maintenance of health" (p. 14). West (1990) thought it imperative that occupational therapists remember that

> age-appropriate, interest-motivating, and self-actualizing occupations abound in everyday play and work environments. These occupations are infinitely better suited to meeting human needs to be accepted, to be useful, and to know the dignity of independence than are all the heat, light, water, electricity, and other physical agents in the world. (p. 9)

Englehardt (1977) claimed that

> Occupational therapy makes a special contribution to our understanding of the importance and the value of human enterprise whereby humans adapt and thrive in their environments by structuring their time in tasks.... In viewing humans as engaged in activities, realizing themselves through their occupation, occupational therapy supports a view of the whole person in function and adaptation.... The virtue of occupational therapy is engagement in the world. (p. 672)

Yerxa et al. (1989) wrote,

> Occupation is a complex phenomenon which is highly individualized and which occurs in an environment in the stream of time.... Occupation provides opportunities for individuals to experience flow, make contributions to selves and others, and discover sociocultural and spiritual meaning through their own actions. (p. 10)

Clark et al. (1991) commented,

> In our practice, we have maintained that what our patients do really matters—it influences their health, their self-respect and their sense of dignity. But we have also declared that it is not so much what they do that is critical as is the acknowledgment that occupation is always pregnant with meaning. Occupation is a uniquely human enterprise because of the extent of its symbolic action. (p. 301)

4. Since World War I, the occupational therapy profession has been perceived as part of the health care system, yet even the founders saw a broader scope for the use of occupational therapy with persons who are well.

The use of occupational therapy for wellness in addition to disability has historical roots. Dunton (as cited in Peloquin, 1991b) stated in 1919 that

> every human being should have both physical and mental occupation. That all should have occupations which they enjoy. These are more necessary when the vocation is dull or distasteful. Every individual should have at least two hobbies, one outdoor and one indoor. A greater number will create wider interests, a greater intelligence. (p. 734)

Hall (as cited in Peloquin, 1991b) called for occupational therapy to be used for healthy people who may lack depth in their lives. Peloquin (1991b) interpreted Dunton's statement to indicate support for occupation in wellness as a creed of our early founders. Later, West (1969) and Johnson (1986) advocated that occupational therapy practitioners be actively involved in preventive health in their communities. Both saw occupation as providing a link to maintaining health and enhancing the quality of people's lives.

Summary

Four core ideas of the occupational therapy profession framed the design of the Lifestyle Redesign Program.

1. Occupation is life itself.
2. Occupation can create new visions of possible selves.
3. Occupation has a curative effect on physical and mental health and on a sense of life order and routine.
4. Occupation has a place in preventive care.

As lifestyle redesigners, occupational therapy practitioners help elderly persons to alter their daily routines so that they can stay healthy and productive and envision new futures. In the following section, we describe concepts from occupational science that informed the design of the Lifestyle Redesign Program and provide vignettes to illustrate these concepts.

Occupational Science

The Lifestyle Redesign Program was designed through the application of occupational science theory and research. *Occupational science* is defined as the systematic "study of the form, function, and meaning of occupation" (Clark, Wood, & Larson, 1998, p. 13). *Occupations* are defined as "the daily activities that can be named in the lexicon of the culture" (Clark et al., 1998, p. 13). Although some occupations are culturally and personally meaningful, others may be boring or virtually meaningless to the person engaged in them. It is therefore essential in thinking about occupation to conceive it as highly personalized. The Lifestyle Redesign Program was shaped by the following perspectives that are studied in occupational science.

Occupation as an Emergent Phenomenon of Transformation

In conceiving the Lifestyle Redesign Program, we recognized the dynamic and generative quality of occupations. Occupations have an "unfolding" nature that is influenced by the person and the setting. Each person brings to the setting his or her emotional makeup, personally defined systems of meaning, and symbolic experiences molded over time. Occupations are created in particular ways and are individualized because of the interaction between the person and the setting during a specific moment in time. This generative quality has the potential to transform the person, the environment, and the larger sociocultural order (Jackson, Carlson, Mandel, Zemke, & Clark, 1998). The following vignette depicts the emergent character of occupation.

> Carmen and Mabel established a personal friendship through their small group interactions in the Lifestyle Redesign Program. Carmen was a Hispanic senior who had always been single. She took pride in her independence and frequently ventured into the community alone to accomplish tasks. However, she yearned for more relationships in her life. Mabel, a Filipino woman, lived with her husband, who spent most of his time at home. Although she expressed a spirit of adventure, she did not have the confidence, knowledge, or skills to attempt unfamiliar trips into the surrounding neighborhood. Together, Carmen and Mabel planned practical outings to places of shared interest.
>
> For example, they took the bus to a store that was familiar to Carmen but new to Mabel. The women encountered a unique, evolving experience with a shared occupation. Carmen added a relationship to her life. This social context was created through her choice to mentor and welcome a

friend. Mabel, in turn, relished the idea of having the freedom to explore her community within the safety of companionship. Her husband did not have the strength to take that risk with her, but Carmen led the way with flair.

In this vignette, we witness how two elderly persons, Carmen and Mabel, combine their daily practices, their understanding of the world, and their personal sense of meaning within the context of a dynamic city environment. Through an ordinary occupation, two people are able to construct occupations that satisfy previously unmet needs and, in the long term, create better health and lifestyle satisfaction.

Meaning

The Lifestyle Redesign Program recognizes that all occupations are not equally meaningful and can vary greatly in their degree of meaningfulness, depending on the person performing the occupation. The extent to which an occupation will be more or less meaningful or important to a person is contingent on his or her values, hopes, experiences, objectives, and life narratives.

On one level, an occupation could be meaningful simply because it created a positive experience, as is the case when one experiences flow (Csikszentmihalyi, 1990) or pleasure. For elderly persons, occupations that evoked feelings of risk were often highly meaningful. The following vignette illustrates risk taking in a meaningful occupation.

> "It's not a lot of planning. It's not long distance. But it's more than they've ever done in terms of trying out a new program." These were the words documented by a leader regarding one of her Lifestyle Redesign Programs groups. The group was nearing the end of their 9-month program, and she was preparing the participants for an independent outing without the occupational therapist.
>
> Plans had to be thorough and precise for the participants to be comfortable enough to even attempt the activity. The group decided to attend a vaudeville musical performance to be held at their retirement home. The outing appeared simple at first; however, the group soon identified major obstacles that would cause them to abandon the activity before participation in the program. The performance was scheduled to take place in the north building, which required many of the participants located in the east building to cross the street. Most critically, the event was held at night, when many of the residents dared not leave their buildings.
>
> This outing required intensive planning and teamwork on the part of the participants to accomplish what some may consider a simple task. With the facilitation of the occupational therapist, they developed a strategy. The group members from the east building would gather together in the

lobby at a designated time. Together, they would cross the street in anticipation of finding Doris, a north building resident, waiting at the door to let them in 15 minutes before show time. For some unexpected reason, if Doris was not there, they would initiate their backup plan. They could call Diana, another north building resident, on the intercom, and she would be in her apartment ready for the signal.

Meanwhile, participants in the north building would commence action to address a different kind of challenge. Designated participants would call those group members with memory impairments. By calling them no more than 30 minutes before the show, they could prompt these members to head downstairs to join the rest of the group.

The participants did just as they planned, although they did add one creative additional factor. The group from the east building brought along their flashlights as they crossed the street. The only social snag was the unexpected $1 donation collected for the musical performance. Although unprepared for the donation, the rest of the plan worked smoothly and safely.

As they processed the experience afterward, the Lifestyle Redesign group members were amazed and proud of their accomplishments. It was an empowering moment when they realized that they were able to network and plan to go to an event as an independent group. They recognized the value of community and how much they relied on their new friends.

Taking risks was memorable for the participants. In this vignette, they experienced excitement and pride in their ability to cross the street and attend the music performance. The Lifestyle Redesign Program had provided the support, education, and experience to boost their confidence to try something new and embed in their memory that they are still risk takers.

Throughout their lives, people embrace "global themes" of meaning, which are convictions or ideologies that become embedded in occupations. "Themes of meaning often guide the manner in which occupations are chosen and performed. Themes of meaning may help people organize their overall everyday pattern of occupation or may provide a framework for interpreting certain occupations as particularly salient or satisfying within the broad context of their lives" (Jackson et al., 1998, p. 328). Common themes of meaning identified among elderly persons included spirituality, family nurturing, or a need to feel useful. The following vignette illustrates how a global theme of meaning can unobtrusively structure how an everyday occupation is enacted.

Mimi was a woman 74 years of age in one of the multiethnic Lifestyle Redesign Program groups. She volunteered to arrive early before group started to set up refreshments. For Mimi, family was an important theme of meaning in her life.

This became evident when she arranged the paper plates, napkins, and utensils in a family format instead of leaving the supplies in organized piles in the traditional buffet style.

The theme of family guided Mimi's actions and was exhibited in the dinner place settings. She expressed her experience in the group as she created a family atmosphere by carefully preparing for the arrival of each anticipated group member. In essence, Mimi's particular practice was socially constructing a "family."

Life narratives provide another context for understanding meaning. Although life events occur as somewhat independent happenings, persons provide coherence to those events by creating narratives. Making sense of events within the framework of a whole story enables persons to experience their lives as moving forward. Life narratives are an evolving process refashioned against the background of new challenges or sociocultural changes. For this reason, persons continually engage in creating and revising their life narratives.

Often it is assumed that elderly persons are engaged solely in life review that creates the final story about their major experiences. However, it is important to remember that elderly persons are still in the process of living, and they, too, can have a sense of forward progression in their life story. In the Lifestyle Redesign Program, narratives were used in two ways. First, occupational storytelling (Clark, Ennevor, & Richardson, 1996) and occupational storymaking were central to the process of the group (an idea that is expanded in chapter 4). Second, each participant was invited to be involved in the making of his or her personal Life History Video (see Appendix 2).

Dynamic Systems Theory

Dynamic systems theory posits that people have the "potential to reorder their patterns of occupations from states of disequilibrium to more complex, stable patterns" (Jackson et al., 1998, p. 328). The Lifestyle Redesign Program used this framework for interpreting patterns of change and stability in human occupations. The designed protocol did not offer a fixed set of occupations "guaranteed" to enhance health and well-being; rather, it provided knowledge and facilitated experiences that allowed participants greater insight into their occupational choices. From there, the participants were encouraged to recognize the potential for an improved quality of life and to identify multiple variables that could bring about lasting changes unique to their life situation (Jackson et al., 1998). In short, they were supported in the development and enactment of a personalized plan of lifestyle redesign. The following vignette illustrates how dynamic systems theory can shed light on the therapeutic process.

> Laura, one of the occupational therapists, described a man in her group who was charming but disruptive. "Roland barrels through the door, interrupting whatever is going on, talking at the top of his voice about some sexual problem with his girlfriend." In individual sessions, Laura came to know Roland as an artist who was intensely searching for clues on how to connect with the world and build successful relationships. She learned that Roland had been mostly deaf since he was a child. Until 74 years of age, he had second-hand hearing aids, which either did not work well or were inappropriate. This explained his sometimes difficult-to-understand speech, his inattention to group discussions, his loud voice, and his interrupting. As Laura worked with Roland, she discovered the many ways that his hearing impairment had shaped and affected his life in dramatic ways.
>
> One day when Roland bemoaned the fact that his car was not working, Laura suggested that he take a public bus to the store to buy art supplies. Laura was surprised by the response from this apparently adventuresome man. "No, no, no! I do not take the bus. Nope, can't do that." With some prodding for the reason, Roland exclaimed, "How do you know when to get off? You could end up anywhere." When Laura suggested that he ask the bus driver, Roland said, "Can't ask questions; you ask questions, and they think you're stupid. I learned that when I was little."
>
> Laura tucked this information away until Roland's group planned their next outing to a museum. Each group member took on some responsibility for the trip. Laura managed to persuade Roland to be in charge of planning the transportation and asking questions, if needed, once they were in the community. On the day of the outing, Roland climbed on the bus, and in his slightly too-loud voice spoke to the bus driver, "We're going to the Natural History Museum, okay?" The bus driver nodded his head.
>
> Weeks later, after several outings via public buses and the underground train, Roland told Laura how she had bolstered him with courage. "I gotta thank you, you know. You've really helped me. I can talk to people now." She was confused because Roland talked all the time. What did he mean? "I mean that I can talk to the big guys. I walk right up and talk to that big guy, you know, the head of this place."

Roland's story is an example of dynamic system change. His life had a stable pattern that was limited by hearing loss and fear of ridicule. Both of these elements had affected his relationships. When he finally arrived at a point in his life where he wanted to learn how to have successful relationships, his usual ways of interacting were inadequate. The "Roland System" was in disequilibrium. In the Lifestyle Redesign Program, Roland

learned some tools, but, more importantly, he overcame some "stuck" places in his life.

The changes came about in what seems to be a small part of Roland's life. He was afraid to ask for directions on a bus. However, this shift had complex effects that radiated throughout his life. Not only did he become a regular bus rider, opening up a new world to him, but he likewise pursued getting a proper hearing aid and started going to dances to meet women. After participating in the Lifestyle Redesign Program, Roland became an urban traveler and even gained the self-confidence to talk to the administrator of his retirement facility.

View of the Human as an Occupational Being

Occupational science embraces the belief that

> it is through one's immersion in the world of occupations that new discoveries about one's potential and a forward movement of one's life takes place. Fear of immersion in occupation can lead to stagnated lives. When fear becomes overwhelming, people remain uncomfortable and stuck in their situation, not able to move forward in life. (Jackson et al., 1998, p. 329)

The USC Well Elderly Study participants were educated regarding the power of ordinary occupations to shape their lives and thereby enhance health and well-being. "The program prepared the participants as 'reflective individuals' (Giddens, 1991) who . . . possessed the tools to consciously recognize their options and overcome fears, make choices that promote health, and experience meaning and satisfaction in their daily routines" (Jackson et al., 1998, p. 329). The participants learned to balance their activities, enact healthy decisions in their lives, and face fears that create stagnation by challenging themselves within a group setting under the care of an occupational therapist. In other words, the participants learned and adopted a process of lifestyle redesign.

Readers may have noticed that these vignettes may exemplify more than one principle. In this last vignette, we see how all of these principles are woven throughout a single life story.

> Clara was a single mother. She raised her daughter on her own and without a high school education. She would sit out on the promenade every afternoon with a group of her friends, visiting and crocheting. She once said, "You have to get up and get dressed and get out. If you just stay in your apartment, you'll die."

As social and assertive as she seemed to be, Clara was shy about trying new things. Her daughter lived halfway across the country and was concerned about her mother falling. Clara was overweight, and she had arthritis and diabetes. At her daughter's suggestion, Clara had not been using steps for more than 2 years. When Clara's group decided that one of their outings should be to take the light-rail train to a farmers' market and craft fair that was at least an hour away, Clara nearly shouted, "Oh no, you're not going to get me on that thing that goes underground." But as the group talked more about the outing for the next 2 weeks, and the occupational therapist outlined the specific steps that would get the group there, Clara was cautiously swayed.

At the end of the train line that day, the group exited the train onto a platform that had eight steps. As Clara carefully made her way down, she stopped halfway and called out, "Hey, somebody take a picture. I'm going down stairs!" At the market, Clara became tired and had to sit down and never made it all the way through. The occupational therapist worried that this outing was going to end up being too taxing for Clara and not a success.

Several months later, the USC Well Elderly team invited Clara to be part of their presentation at the state conference for occupational therapy practitioners. Clara decided to tell the story of the outing day.

"When we went back on the train, some of the elevators were closed. There were escalators—I haven't been on an escalator in 9 or 10 years. One of the other members kept saying, 'Come on, come on.' Then one person took one of my arms, someone took my walker, and someone else was behind me. Then someone counted 'One, two, three.' It was like they carried me down that escalator. They made me do it. They said I could do it, and I did do it. That day, I did two things I thought I never would do. That night, when I thought about it, I thought that when people have faith in you, and they say you can do it, you can!"

After her group had ended, Clara was one of the residents in her building who decided that they would try to enter the Los Angeles Marathon. They were planning on having a group of people with walkers to follow the wheelchair racers. Clara was the only resident who actually did it. The day of the marathon, it was raining in Los Angeles, a steady drizzle. By 6:30 a.m., Clara jostled her way through the crowds of thousands and waited for her time to start. The bicycles went, then the wheelchairs, then the runners began. She waded into the edge of the throng, and she was off. By the time Clara had walked a half of a mile, all of the other participants were nowhere to be seen, and the street sweepers were starting to cleanup. Her friend held an umbrella over her head and wondered if Clara really wanted to do more. Yes, she wanted to go on. Clara has a photo of herself, at 77 years of age, standing with her walker, arms raised in victory, under the 1 mile marker of the race.

Clara brought a strong sense of self-reliance and determination to her experience in the Lifestyle Redesign Program. She additionally brought fears and anxieties about moving beyond the predictable areas of her apartment and the promenade. From her interactions with the other group members and the occupational therapist, Clara realized that she was drawn to occupations that were adventurous. Taking the first risks on that train ride changed the way that Clara saw herself. It was almost as if Clara became that train. Would she come and make a speech to a group of professionals? "I've never given a speech before, but sure, why not?" Participate in the marathon? "Why not?" She knew the importance of getting out of her apartment everyday, she just did not know how far she could go. "Getting out" now took on a new meaning for Clara.

In her speech, Clara credited the occupational therapist for her own accomplishments. "The leaders are so strong—they say lean on me, and I do what they say." But Clara, the therapist, the group, the environment—they were all systems that were dynamically interacting. No one could have predicted the way that train ride would affect Clara, that she would radiate vitality throughout the rest of her life. Because she was too tired to see all of the market that day, was the outing an unsuccessful intervention for Clara? She did not think so.

In this chapter, we have highlighted the foundational concepts of the Lifestyle Redesign Program. However, implications of this program must be customized for local settings. In chapter 3, we provide guidelines for how to conduct a needs evaluation practically and efficiently in other settings. ■

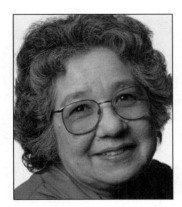

3

Needs Evaluation

Just as an occupational therapy evaluation is the foundation for client treatment, a needs evaluation provides critical information for the planning process of service providers and other decision makers and planners (Billings & Cowley, 1995; Polit & Hungler, 1991). Needs evaluation leads to clear objectives (Roberts, 1996), which allow for more effective therapeutic interventions and outcomes. Krupnick (1996) stated, "As professionals within a large health care system, occupational therapy practitioners must be able to assess their audience and adjust their message for particular target groups" (p. 118).

What Is a Needs Evaluation?

Needs evaluations, which provide information for action, serve a useful purpose before and after a service program is in operation (Polit & Hungler, 1991). A needs evaluation is a systematic investigation of the needs of a group, community, or organization for specific services or policies (Kniepmann, 1997; Polit & Hungler, 1991). Information is gathered regarding the strengths, problems, resources, and barriers in a given population or community (Kniepmann, 1997).

The type of needs uncovered depends on the perspective of the evaluator. For example, sociologists have adopted Bradshaw's taxonomy (as cited in Billings & Cowley, 1995) of formative need, felt need, expressed need, and comparative need. A distinction is made between the needs as identified by the professional and those "felt" by the person.

The traditional epidemiologist uses community morbidity and mortality data to prioritize the allocation of public health resources (Ashley & McLachlan, as cited in Billings & Cowley, 1995; Knox, as cited in Billings & Cowley, 1995). The needs of the community are noted, but the persons themselves do not confirm the findings.

The health economist defines *need* according to cost effectiveness and supply and demand. Areas of need are considered relative and "can be 'traded off' against each other, given limited resources" (Billings & Cowley, 1995, p. 722).

Occupational therapy practitioners are most concerned with the needs, desires, and goals as perceived and recognized by individual clients. Although the focus is on a therapeutic, occupation-centered process, pragmatism forces a consideration of cost effectiveness.

Various needs evaluation strategies have strengths and weaknesses. The setting being evaluated and other conditions will demand an appropriate strategy. Some qualities of various needs evaluation strategies are listed in Table 1.

In addition to collecting critical information, the process of evaluating needs may be an opportunity for building respect and rapport within the community for which a program is designed. By requesting a person's insight and feedback, the client's perspective is validated.

Qualitative Approaches

We believe that a qualitative approach to needs evaluation is one of the most powerful ways to truly comprehend and address the unique needs of a group of clients in a Lifestyle Redesign Program. However, we must clarify that we do not expect practitioners to conduct a full-blown qualitative research study as a needs evaluation before implementing the Lifestyle Redesign Program. Instead, we suggest they adapt qualitative methods so that they are clinically feasible.

Collecting Rich Descriptions

Qualitative researchers strive to acquire a complex understanding of the participants' physical and social worlds. When attempting to enhance health and well-being or to help an elderly person to remain independent in the community, one must look at the myriad issues that could be creating stress or compromising health. For example, staying in one's home could be due to mobility problems that could be easily corrected with adaptive equipment. However, with further discussion, the practitioner may find that fear about safety and lack of companionship for daily excursions contribute more to being isolated than do typical mobility problems. Rich descriptions that take into account the various factors that influence the problems and strengths of elderly persons can be collected through interviews.

Capturing the Subjective Meaning of Occupations

Perceived health, happiness, and life satisfaction to some extent depend on each person's vision about what constitutes a quality life. One's upbringing, social status, possessions, degree of control, religious affiliations, and personal attitude toward life are among the many factors that determine one's health and receptivity to occupations in older adulthood. Therefore, for the Lifestyle Redesign Program to be effective, the therapists need to have insight into the meaning the elderly persons attribute to their occupations. Interviewing enables the therapist to obtain a complete, in-depth picture of the

Table 1
Approaches to Needs Evaluation

Type	Description	Examples
Focus groups or community forum	Group of people Facilitator led Open-ended questions	Consumers
Key informant	Individual interview Interviewee who is aware of the needs of the target group Open-ended questions	Housing directors Senior club members Facility staff members Residents
Survey	Data collected from a sample of the target group Closed-ended or semistructured questions	Population census
Indicators or community profiling	From statistics available in existing records	Census bureau Police records
Literature review	Information from recent publications	Journals Books Articles

Note. Adapted from needs evaluation approaches by Billings and Cowley (1995), Kniepmann (1997), and Polit and Hungler (1991).

person's story of himself or herself as an occupational being, including which occupations are or have the potential to be deeply meaningful.

Claiming Everyday Experiences

Qualitative researchers are typically concerned with everyday experiences (i.e., the naturally occurring events that take place in the environments in which persons find themselves). Occupations are of central concern to occupational therapy practitioners and are among the class of events on which qualitative research has typically focused. For this reason, qualitative interviewing is a useful method for occupational therapy practitioners to obtain essential information. This information may include the finer details about daily occupations, the social or cultural context in which occupations occur, companionship that accompanies occupation, the social personal timing of occupations, and the risks involved in occupation. Each of these concerns can be formulated as a question for the needs evaluation interview.

In most cases, evaluating needs will involve conducting individualized interviews on concerns related to the Lifestyle Redesign Program and then making sense of them through clinical reasoning rather than through the coding of transcripts of tape-recorded interviews. See Box 4 for helpful guidelines to conduct qualitative needs evaluations.

Individual Interviews

In an upcoming section, we describe the interview process and list the core questions that were used in the needs evaluation of the USC Well Elderly Study. Some additional questions for guiding the needs evaluation interview are listed.

- What do you do each day?
- What do you believe are the barriers to doing what you would like to do each day?
- What things that you do are particularly meaningful?
- What special issues in daily living are bothering you right now? What creates stress in your life?
- What do you think is essential for a quality life?
- Throughout life, people choose to do certain activities they love. Can you describe the activities that have been most important in your life at each period, beginning with childhood and up to the present?
- What is it about these activities that you most like to do? What makes them attractive to you?

- Do you have daily routines or habits? How important is routine in your life?
- What aspects of aging have you found the most challenging?
- If you could change anything in your situation, what would you change?

Occupational therapists may of course add other questions.

Focus Groups

Focus groups, one of the newer methods used in qualitative research (Morgan, 1997), aim to gather valuable information about a particular topic through input generated by a group of persons with the guidance of a moderator. Focus groups have been used for many purposes (Templeton, 1987), but we believe they are particularly

Box 4
Guidelines for
Qualitative Needs Evaluations

Needs evaluations using individual interviews will be performed in different ways; however, these are a few guidelines to consider.

- Use an outside therapist when collecting the data so that residents feel free to share information.
- Tape recording requires a judgment call. Although tape recording can be intimidating to the resident, it is virtually impossible to remember or write down all the nuances of information that are often an essential key to programming. In every situation, we have tape recorded without a problem and, in fact, have found recording to be a great advantage. However, tape recording is not strictly necessary, and good note taking and clinical reasoning may be used in its place.
- It is important to use an additive or iterative approach. In other words, determine a time when the group of therapists collecting the data can reflect on their findings, clarify those findings with other therapists, and revise the interview protocol. The development of the interview protocol is an emerging process. Insights gained from 1 day of interviews should be used to restructure the interview on the following day.

useful in the exploratory stages of implementing the Lifestyle Redesign Program in local settings. These groups often stimulate production of creative concepts, generate impressions about programs, identify or diagnose problems, and uncover underlying attitudes about living situations. To implement the Lifestyle Redesign Program, questions such as those suggested earlier can be modified for a group response or used verbatim in the group process when appropriate.

There are many advantages to using focus groups as part of a needs evaluation before implementing the Lifestyle Redesign Program. Focus groups validate the participants by making them a part of an informant group. The participant may feel privileged to be able to provide input in the initial stages of program development. "Respect is particularly important when approaching individuals in the community.... Respect includes an appreciation for their perspective—what is in this for them—a valuable question to consider" (Roberts, 1996, p. 1260). The dynamic process of a focus group allows participants to be stimulated by and build on each others' ideas and generate concepts that may have remained uncovered in individual interviews (Stewart & Shamdasani, 1990). Focus groups are flexible and often explore unanticipated areas, new questions, and a broader range of information, insight, and ideas (Coyne & Calarco, 1995; Lautar, 1996; Millar, Maggs, Warner, & Whale, 1996).

> The open response format of a focus group provides an opportunity to obtain large and rich amounts of data in the respondents' own words. The researcher can obtain deeper levels of meaning, make important connections, and identify subtle nuances in expression and meaning. (Stewart & Shamdasani, 1990, p. 16)

Focus groups allow the researcher the opportunity to clarify responses directly and to probe other members for contradictory or similar ideas. Discussing different perspectives on a topic can uncover deeper issues that can then be addressed or identify diverse ideas that may need to be incorporated into planning a program. Focus groups are cost-effective ways to acquire more information within a specific time period than individual interviews.

Although focus groups have many advantages, they likewise have disadvantages that must be considered. One disadvantage is that some persons are too shy to be open in a group context; these participants should be interviewed individually. A second disadvantage is that

one vociferous or opinionated person may bias or dominate the group process. Finally, the group leader, because of his or her position, runs the risk of biasing the results and must be trained in how to avoid this possibility.

The following are some suggested questions for focus groups.

- Why would someone want to live in this retirement home?
- What makes this residence unique?
- Why do people leave this retirement home?
- What programs and activities are offered here? Which do you recommend and why?
- How active are the residents here?
- What are the differences between independent, assisted, and nursing care living?
- What modes of transportation do you use?
- Where do you go in the neighboring communities?
- Where would you like to go?
- What stressors or obstacles do you face as a retiree?
- What would you like to see changed in your community? Retirement home? Apartment?
- What are the most meaningful activities that fill your time?
- How would you like to use your time better?
- If there were one thing you could add to your life, what would it be?
- What would you like to learn regarding your health and wellness?

In the next section, we present three examples, varying in rigor, of needs evaluations that we have used in setting up the Lifestyle Redesign Program.

Examples of Needs Evaluation

The USC Well Elderly Study

The needs evaluation for the USC Well Elderly Study (Clark et al., 1996) was an extensive project to gain information about what elderly persons perceived were important areas of activity and the strategies of adaptation they used to achieve life satisfaction. The information was then used in developing the Lifestyle Redesign Program protocol.

Data collection began when USC Well Elderly Study research assistants conducted semistructured interviews with 29 elderly persons who lived at the site. Of the 29 participants, 20 were women, and 9 were men. Participants were from the following ethnic backgrounds: African-American (2), Asian-American (1), white (20), and Hispanic (6). The research assistants conducted an audiotaped one-on-one interview with each respondent that lasted between 1 and 2 hr. Five questions prompted the participant to share information about his or her needs and adaptations. Questions of this nature may be included in interviews and focus groups for needs evaluations at other sites.

1. Tell me about your life at Angelus Plaza?
2. Do you like living here? Why or why not, and what do or do not like about it?
3. What do you do every day to stay happy and healthy?
4. What is different about living here compared with other situations in which you have lived?
5. Why do people leave Angelus Plaza?

Each researcher asked the above questions and then supplemented the interview with questions on the basis of information provided by previous interviewees. This is referred to as the *method of naturalistic inquiry* (see Lincoln & Guba, 1981).

Four steps were used to analyze the data. First, each researcher generated a summary of the content of each interview and recorded any statements that suggested an adaptive strategy on a note card. Second, each researcher developed a typology of life domains from the content of the interviews. Third, a senior investigator then interviewed each of the researchers about their typology by using the method described by Lincoln and Guba (1981). This resulted in a single typology of life domains that was confirmed as accurate by the entire research team. Fourth, another set of researchers refined the categories of the typology through hermeneutic dialogue and reasoning. The concrete product of this labor-intensive process was a 10-step typology. At this point, steps 2 and 4 were repeated to ascertain the adaptive strategies under each life domain. Some of these life domains and adaptive strategies were used as modules for the Lifestyle Redesign Program.

In the following sections, we describe two less rigorous approaches to needs evaluation that we have used in implementing the Lifestyle Redesign Program.

The Arizona Project

Casa Maria is a small retirement establishment that consists of three levels of care. Town homes and apartments are available for residents who want community living with housekeeping assistance. Essentially, residents at

this level consider themselves independent community dwellers. The second level of care is assisted living, and the third level of care is a skilled nursing facility for persons who need 24-hr care and medical support. Our task was to perform a needs evaluation and design a program for residents in the second level of care, assisted living.

The most efficient approach for quickly completing the needs evaluation phase was to have 3 therapists spend 2 days interviewing the 12 residents who would be included in the program. It is important to note that interviewing all the potential participants in a proposed program is not necessary and was not done for the USC Well Elderly Study. However, in this case, because of the small number of residents scheduled to take part in the Lifestyle Redesign Program, 3 therapists could complete the entire project in 2 days. Additionally, we interviewed the staff members to obtain their viewpoints about the needs of the residents.

One of the 2 therapists was responsible for interviewing the staff members. The other 2 therapists each interviewed 1 person in the morning by using the 5 questions presented above as a guideline. Each therapist then wrote a summary of the content from the tape-recorded interview and identified possible areas of concern that were defined as domains of need on which the program should focus. This procedure was repeated in the afternoon. That evening, the 3 therapists met to share the identified areas of concern. On the basis of a compilation and clarification of all the areas of concern, the practitioners added new questions to the interview protocol for subsequent interviews.

For example, if a therapist found from her interview of a respondent that privacy was an issue that interfered with life satisfaction, then a question concerning privacy was added to the interview prompts. The following day, each therapist used the revised interview with 2 residents—1 in the morning and 1 in the afternoon. By the second day, all residents and staff members had completed the process. The therapists then engaged in a 2-hr dialog in which they fleshed out and prioritized the areas of concern. This information was discussed with the occupational therapist based at the facility, and the program was thus developed.

The Pomona Project

San Gabriel Villas is a retirement community with the same structure as Casa Maria. There is continuous care for residents from independent living to skilled nursing care.

The focus group format was used to evaluate needs at this site. A presentation to the resident's council informed them about the Lifestyle Redesign Program. After the council approved having the program come to their community, notices were sent out to the residents requesting volunteers to be part of the focus groups. Through a combination of random selection and recommendations by the facility director, 20 residents were selected as representatives of their community.

The facility director assisted in arranging a room and time so that two groups could meet for 2 hr each. Before beginning the first group, each of the 10 participants filled out a brief questionnaire made up of several open-ended questions similar to those that were later posed to the group. This procedure allowed the participants to formulate their own thoughts and opinions.

One therapist acted as the group leader and facilitated a lively discussion about life at San Gabriel Villas by using questions similar to those presented in the previous section. The leader framed questions to include positive aspects of their living environment as well as soliciting concerns or issues. A second therapist took notes and acted as an observer of the interactions. She was able to cue the leader when it appeared a group member had something to add to the discussion. The focus group was audiotaped. The recording served as a reference to confirm the themes and ideas that were generated in the discussion.

After reviewing the initial focus group feedback, we returned for our second and final focus group. This second group included new volunteers as well as those residents who were willing and able to return. This meeting consisted of more participants and was 1 hr in length. Our goal was to confirm and refine an understanding of the needs that were identified previously.

In addition, representatives from administration, rehabilitation staff members, and maintenance staff members were informally interviewed. They were asked to share their perspectives on the culture of this community and available resources. When these data were combined with that of the focus groups, the synthesis provided sufficient information to adapt the Lifestyle Redesign Program for this new location in a relatively short time and in a cost-effective manner.

Once the needs evaluation is conducted, the findings are used to modify the Lifestyle Redesign Program for implementation in the local setting. In chapter 4, we specify the methods of delivery that must be retained in every Lifestyle Redesign Program. ■

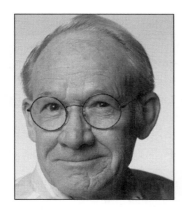

4

Methods of Delivery

I n the Lifestyle Redesign Program used in the USC Well Elderly Study, both group and individual formats were used for therapeutic sessions. This decision to combine both formats was made on the basis of occupational therapy literature that supports benefits from each method that are different and yet supportive of each other (Carlson, Fanchiang, Zemke, & Clark, 1996). In this section, we will examine elements of group treatment, what the Lifestyle Redesign Program groups were like, and how they differed from other models of group interventions.

Groups

Throughout the history of occupational therapy, clients have been treated in groups. Over time, the emphasis of group work has changed and has included project completion, ego building, and social adaptation (Schwartzberg, 1998). Today, occupational therapy practitioners use various approaches to group work in various settings. Some of these are task groups, range-of-motion groups, activity groups, cooking groups, sensorimotor groups, or peer support groups. As with psychotherapy groups, success is determined in part by the leader's understanding of and facility with theories of group process and group dynamics.

Group work is both exciting and complex because the leader must simultaneously foster the growth of the group identity and cohesiveness while remembering the goals for change of individual members. In fostering a group, some of the considerations of the leader include which phase the group is operating; how comfortable the members are with the leader and one another; how cohesive the group is; and the skills, personalities, and challenges that individual members contribute to dynamic interactions. In general, occupational therapy groups focus more on *doing,* whereas psychotherapy groups rely on talking as an interactive medium.

Although we know that our readers have had training in this area through their occupational therapy education, inclusion of the material serves as a reminder that the Lifestyle Redesign Program is not simply an educational program but is a deeply therapeutic process. Occupational therapists leading the groups must therefore harness their skills in therapeutic group work. A few of the general principles of group process that we believe are particularly helpful to leading Lifestyle Redesign Program groups are described below. Our hope is that, before implementing the Lifestyle Redesign Program, therapists will review at least one of the references we have cited.

Practitioner textbooks (Bender, Norris, & Bauckham, 1991; Borg & Bruce, 1991; Brown, 1988; Bruce &

Borg, 1993; Burnside, 1978; Cole, 1998; Howe & Schwartzberg, 1995; Toseland, 1995) describe the elements of the group therapy process in various ways. They address group dynamics, the therapeutic relationship, types of groups, how to begin a group, and how to end one. Toseland (1995) classified the skills required of a group leader as follows.

- Facilitation: engaging, clarifying, responding
- Data gathering and evaluation: identifying, synthesizing
- Action skills: linking, providing resources, modeling

In general, the task of the occupational therapist in such groups is to provide an environment in which persons can change in some way. Furthermore, Toseland (1995) reminded us that it is important to include all participants in the group. He referred to Yalom's concept of

> universalizing a group member's experience. Involving all members helps to identify commonalities in older adults' life experiences. As members become involved, they realize how particular problems affect them and how a solution to one member's problem can be directly or indirectly helpful to them. (as cited in Toseland, 1995, p. 66)

Finally, it should be noted that it is crucial that therapists possess expertise in this area for the Lifestyle Redesign Program to be fully successful. The decision to execute the Lifestyle Redesign Program mainly in groups was made primarily because of the therapeutic benefit of group process and only secondarily because of potential cost benefits. We believe that only through a carefully monitored group process can the therapeutic benefits described in the next section be achieved.

The Structure of the Lifestyle Redesign Program

The goal of the Lifestyle Redesign Program was to increase or maintain the independence, health, and well-being of elderly persons who were living independently. The elderly persons met in their own small groups for 2 hr each week for 9 months. The groups were led by an occupational therapist who offered up to 9 hr of individual interaction to each participant during the course of the program. The weekly, 2-hr group meetings addressed topics that had been previously identified in the needs evaluation described earlier (Clark et al., 1996). Approximately every fourth meeting, the group and the occupational therapist ventured out into the surrounding community so that they could engage in the world in

new ways. Each structured group session was filled with content from 1 of the 9 content modules described in chapter 5. At this point, we focus on the structure and process of the Lifestyle Redesign Program.

Group Sessions

Each elderly person attended a 2-hr meeting each week where he or she encountered the same group of people for 9 months. The meetings were held in a room that was no farther than across the street from where the residents lived. As an elderly person entered the meeting area, he or she would find a central table surrounded by stable chairs. On one side of the room was a tablecloth-covered refreshment area with coffee, lemonade, water, and a selection of teas. Each week, some kind of snack was provided, usually something healthy or novel. Typically, one or more residents would arrive early and help the occupational therapist set up the food and beverages, and others would stay at the end of the meeting to assist with cleanup. Within 15 minutes of the official starting time, the occupational therapist would begin the session.

During the set-up period, participants frequently visited with one another or sought the attention of the occupational therapist to relate recent events in their lives. Sometimes these discussions would become part of the official meeting by being incorporated into topics on occupation and health.

The occupational therapist acted as a leader of the group. According to Bruce and Borg (1993), the role of the occupational therapy therapist as the leader of a group is to ensure safety, foster trust, be congruent, value himself or herself, value the client, foster open communication, value change, accept tentativeness, and provide limits and boundaries. He or she would describe what the group was going to discuss that day. In the meeting's most formal format, the occupational therapist would begin by introducing a subject and promote discussion by posing questions highlighting the occupational aspect of the topic. For example, "How do transportation resources and constraints affect one's occupational choices?" (Jackson, Carlson, Mandel, Zemke, & Clark, 1998, p. 335). The occupational therapist would ground the discussion with examples from his or her own life and then solicit similar responses from each participant. He or she would then move the discussion to a consideration of the way in which occupations shape one's use of transportation options. Individual concerns would be aired through this discussion, and one or more of the participants or the occupational therapist would offer solutions, insights, commiseration, or even challenges in response.

During the discussion, the occupational therapist or one of the participants would often list the ideas on a large flip chart. At this meeting or the next, the occupational therapist would lead the discussion toward the idea of doing something as a group that was related to the topic, such as trying out a form of transportation that was new to most of the participants. Together, the group would brainstorm about what they wanted to do. The occupational therapist would shape the discussion to include consideration of what was practically entailed in any event and foster problem solving of any constraints. Often, the occupational therapist would offer suggestions for activities to broaden the choice of options that might be possible. Most of the outings were inexpensive, and the program paid for all basic costs.

Outside of the meeting time, the occupational therapist or one of the participants would research various aspects of a plan, sometimes even visiting the site to evaluate accessibility or make arrangements for accommodations. The evening before an outing, a special reminder would be placed under the door of each participant's apartment. These notices would include pertinent reminders, such as to wear comfortable shoes or bring reading glasses. The occupational therapist brought water and cups, some form of sugar, some small snack foods, and information on each participant, including medical coverage and next of kin on each outing. Usually the occupational therapist or one of the participants would take photographs. In the meeting after an outing, the therapist would initiate a discussion about the outing to prompt the participants to engage in a self-reflective process regarding their experience and solicit comments about what was successful or problematic. The therapist would attempt to integrate reflections on the outing experience with the ongoing discussion of occupation.

Individual Sessions

For individual sessions, the occupational therapist usually met with participants in their own apartments. Often a resident would provide tea or coffee, and the occupational therapist would encourage a discussion about the resident's occupations. Asking questions about photographs or knickknacks triggered many stories about family members or friends. Sometimes discussions would focus on events or topics from group meetings or outings. The therapist may have noticed some puzzling

or intriguing response on the part of the resident during a group session and would seize the opportunity to encourage deeper discussion or disclosures that were not likely to happen in the larger group. These one-on-one exchanges allowed the occupational therapist to learn many things about each resident that subsequently could be developed or addressed, not necessarily explicitly, during group sessions (see Appendix 1 for more information about individual sessions).

The Lifestyle Redesign Program as a Transformational Process

The structure of the program interaction, as described above, provided a mix of regularity or sameness and novelty or change. The group sessions met at the same place, time, and day of every week and lasted for the same amount of time. The leader and group members were consistent throughout the 9-month program. The meetings were organized in a routine format. The discussions focused on the concept of occupation and topics that were relevant to the lives of the individual participants. Even special events or outings occurred at regular intervals.

At the same time, the group sessions allowed for variety, spontaneity, and improvisation. Each week, the topic or theme of the meeting changed. Materials were presented in various formats. New ideas and technologies were introduced. Guest speakers provided specialized materials and skills. Snacks would change from one week to the next. The tone of the sessions changed with different activities and over time as participants got to know each other and shared common experiences. In short, the sessions blended predictability and stability with change and growth.

Several techniques were important to the group process. One example was to position group members as experts. From the beginning, it seemed important that each resident was seen and recognized as an expert in many areas. Much of what concerns the practice of occupational therapy is the solving of problems that arise in everyday living. The fact that these elderly persons had lived to their present ages strongly indicated that they had all been successful in solving many of life's challenges. In general, our expectation was that, together, the occupational therapist and each participant would share various solutions and perspectives that would be enriching in two ways. First, information would be offered, much as it is in a classroom. Second, as residents shared their stories and information, they developed greater self-respect and a sense that others valued their perspectives and life knowledge, which seemed to be empowering.

Another technique that seemed to promote the therapeutic process was reproducing selected feedback phrases in a printed format. In the Lifestyle Redesign Program groups, the occupational therapist would lead discussions on various topics (e.g., "What is health?") and solicit responses from each participant on what his or her ideas were. The leader would record these responses onto a large flip chart. The responses were then organized, typed, printed in large fonts, and returned to the participants in a subsequent session. These response sheets would then be assembled as part of a notebook (see Ending a Group in chapter 5) for each resident. These notebooks contained all the group handouts and provided a record of their experiences in the Lifestyle Redesign Program. Seeing one's own words in print seemed to be affirming for the respondents. As a result, they appeared to view themselves as more real, more valid, and more important.

In the following sections, we more broadly address what we did and discuss what we believe happened.

What We Did in the Lifestyle Redesign Program

The model of the USC Well Elderly Study in the second box of Figure 4 (Jackson et al., 1998) includes methods for delivering the Lifestyle Redesign Program content. The categories didactic presentation, peer exchange, direct experience, and personal exploration are listed. Each of the categories is described below.

Didactic Presentation

The didactic presentation is the information that the occupational therapist brought to the group. Three types of materials were offered in what was the closest to a classroom format. These materials included specialized occupational therapy content (e.g., how to conserve energy and protect joints) as well as other kinds of practical information (e.g., the comparative costs of different types of transportation). Furthermore, many sessions focused strictly on occupation or on the process of occupational self-analysis. However, all content was related to occupational concerns.

Didactic presentations on occupation and the process of occupational self-analysis gave the residents a

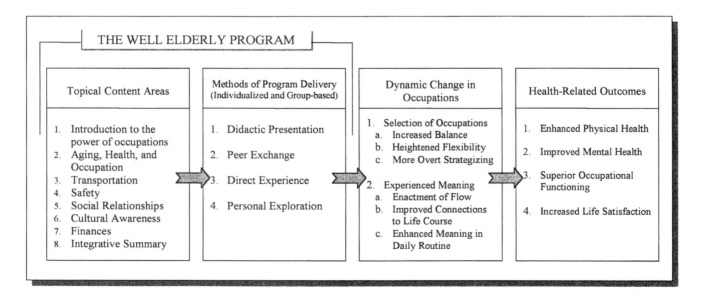

Figure 4. USC Well Elderly program model. From "Occupation in Lifestyle Redesign: The Well Elderly Study Occupational Therapy Program," by J. Jackson, M. Carlson, D. Mandel, R. Zemke, and F. Clark, 1998, *American Journal of Occupational Therapy, 52*, p. 330. Copyright 1998 by the American Occupational Therapy Association. Reprinted with permission.

new way of being in the world, a new standpoint from which to view themselves as agentic persons. Knowledge about occupation and its effect on one's health and life history provided the resident with a new perspective from which to view the self, the world, and their interaction.

Within the didactic sessions, the occupational therapist became a coach, whereas the residents were apprentices of occupational self-analysis. At the moment of presenting information, the occupational therapist and how he or she was presenting it created a model of how to use information. The therapist was modeling a culture of self-reflection and demonstrating a consideration of problem solving.

Peer Exchange

The concept of peer exchange refers to the residents' storytelling in group sessions. They told stories about their lives, how they met challenges, or what they did yesterday. We believe the allocation of session time to such storytelling was critical to the success of the program. Although these stories, on the surface, sometimes appeared mundane, McAdams (as cited in Belenky, Bond, & Weinstock, 1997) argued that storytelling is crucial for creating the self.

> The story is the person's identity. The story provides the person with a sense of unity and purpose in life—a sense that one is a whole being moving forward in a particular direction. From the standpoint of personal identity, therefore, the person is both historian and history—a storyteller who creates the self in the telling. (Belenky et al., 1997, p. 151)

Direct Experience

For an occupational therapist, the term *direct experience* would usually invoke a vision of someone actively doing something. The Lifestyle Redesign Program was infused with as much active doing as possible, an idea that is discussed in greater detail in the next section. At this point, it is useful to think of the program as more of a "doing" therapy than a "talking" therapy with many kinds of doing.

- Doing in one's apartment
- Doing in group sessions
- Doing with therapist support
- Doing on one's own
- Doing in the community
- Doing in one's imagination

We believe that such engagement in the world of activity gave the residents a renewed sense of themselves as agents in their self-regulation and self-organization, as persons more in command of their lives and in control of their time.

Personal Exploration

Time was reserved in group sessions for the residents to reflect on the meaningfulness, or importance, of the didactic content for their lives. Exercises were developed so that they would be assisted in applying the presented concepts to their individual concerns. A selection of these exercises is included in the coverage of the modules in chapter 5.

What Happened in the Lifestyle Redesign Program

Rogers (1980), in his review of his life from 65 to 75 years of age, described his life as dynamic and changing in many ways. He referred to being open to suggestions from others, having a readiness for new ventures, and being "bored by safety and sureness" (Rogers, 1980, p. 77). Yet we sensed that, before their participation in the Lifestyle Redesign Program, many of the elderly persons at the study sites seemed to feel "flat," as if they were "stuck" or stagnating. We believe that, for these persons, the Lifestyle Redesign Program sessions became places of transformation.

Although didactic and structured content was presented in most sessions, a deeply therapeutic process transpired. Through this process (over time and through graduated experience), residents who wanted to be transformed were, in fact, transformed. They found they were eventually able to develop and implement a customized plan of personally meaningful, health-promoting occupation anchored in a daily routine that made it sustainable.

One way in which to describe the process is to talk about it in terms of the following four steps.

1. Acquiring knowledge of the factors related to occupation that promote health and happiness
2. Performing a personal inventory and reflecting on one's fears and occupational choices, interests, life goals, and so forth (occupational self-analysis)
3. Overcoming one's fears by taking incremental risks in the real world of activity in small steps over time
4. Weaving together the outcomes of the prior steps to develop a health-promoting daily routine (Carlson, Clark, & Young, 1998)

We found that even for those residents who were used to a routine or resistant to change (Reich & Zautra, 1991), small steps taken over time generated the courage to overcome fears, experiment with refraining from old habits, and take larger risks. Although, in the case of the USC Well Elderly Study, the Lifestyle Redesign Program was spread over 9 months, it is possible that the outcomes could have been accomplished in less time. However, only future research will be able to verify this claim. In the meantime, we are confident that these positive outcomes can be achieved in the 9-month time frame.

It is interesting that not all the persons who consistently attended the Lifestyle Redesign Program in the USC Well Elderly Study had obvious occupational dysfunctions or problems with sustaining a healthy routine. For one participant who seemed to have no evident limitations, simply experiencing growth and learning was enough to keep her attending regularly. We believe that, at a minimum, the participants learned four key ideas during the therapeutic process that were incorporated into a more general perspective on life. This perspective enabled them to possess a relatively well-articulated, long-term strategy for promoting health and well-being through engagement in occupation.

Key Ideas of the Lifestyle Redesign Program

1. Experience in occupation produces radiating, not linear, change.

Experience is defined as "an activity or practice through which knowledge or skill is gained" (*American Heritage Dictionary*, 1989, p. 248). However, other scholars expand this idea by proposing that it is in the world of experience that growth, learning, and a vital sense of the self arises (Applegate & Bonovitz, 1995; Lave & Wenger, 1991; Rogers, 1980). The Lifestyle Redesign Program heavily incorporates experience in everyday activities of graduated levels of challenge and complexity as a way of creating transformation. Furthermore, the program stresses the ways in which experience (following the principles of dynamic systems theory) could create radiating, not linear, change. For example, venturing out on the newly operating train system for the first time could serve not only as a context for learning transportation skills but also for building a new self-image as an "urban traveler" and for developing a sense of

social connectedness, all of which could ultimately benefit health.

2. Occupational self-analysis is possible.

Although nearly all of the participants had heard of psychoanalysis (a "talking" therapy), virtually none had heard of occupational self-analysis (a largely "doing" therapy). The Lifestyle Redesign Program took the participants through the process slowly, thoughtfully, and experientially. The participants were challenged to reflect on who they were as occupational beings, to think about the occupations that they had always found or were presently finding most fulfilling, and to evaluate the extent to which they were experiencing occupational deprivation or dysfunction. They were encouraged to identify the fears or physical limitations that were barriers to engagement in the world and then determine the small steps they could take to overcome these barriers.

The plans would then be enacted (with the support of the therapist or the group when required). After taking new risks and completing exercises in the modules, the participants were asked to reflect on their experiences and integrate their new understanding into the strategies for lifestyle redesign that they were mastering. Through this process, they began to move from an image of themselves as "I can't anymore" to "I can" (Mandel & Roy, 1995).

3. When people understand the elements of occupation, they have the tool kit to redesign their lives.

Flavell (as cited in Belenky et al., 1997) wrote that

> A person's theory of mind is of the utmost importance. People who are aware of the intellectual tools that they have at their disposal are likely to cultivate and use those tools much more effectively and consistently than are people who have not yet articulated the existence and function of a tool. (p. 58)

The Lifestyle Redesign Program created a new way for the participants to view themselves and conceive of their interactions in the world. It gave them a new way of thinking about their existence and how they spend their time, one that emphasized the "chunks of activities" (occupations) they engaged in each day and how what they chose to do affected their health, happiness, and well-being. In short, they came to see occupation as the fundamental fabric of daily life. Furthermore, they began to appreciate that through conscious reflection they could positively affect their life satisfaction, health, and cognitive functioning. This mindset was grounded in the perspective that remaining engaged in life was a key factor in successful aging, and that each person could learn to redesign his or her lifestyle to be happier and healthier.

The "tool kit" for lifestyle redesign incorporated several key elements in two broad areas: selection style and experienced meaning (Jackson et al., 1998).

Selection style. Lifestyle redesign most fundamentally involves selecting occupations. The participants became familiar with concepts such as balance, routinization, flexibility, orchestration, and time structure that could contribute to the formulation of an overall, well-articulated agenda for promoting health and well-being. We believe that, for this reason, the elderly persons in the Lifestyle Redesign Program were less likely to drift aimlessly in selecting occupations. Their selection style became grounded in an overarching framework for choosing activities.

Experienced meaning. Maslow (1987) and Frankl (1969) are well known for their belief that the ability to find meaning in one's life represents a basic, universal human need. Participants in the Lifestyle Redesign Program were exposed to the multiple dimensions of meaningfulness that emanate from participation in occupation. They learned that occupations could be meaningful by virtue of the degree of flow (Csikszentmihalyi, 1990) they produced; *flow* is defined as the positive psychological state that results when engaged in an occupation in which the challenge carefully matches one's ability level. Second, they learned that occupations could be meaningful because they were tied to one's past history but could likewise be judged as worthwhile because of their connection to the present. Finally, the participants learned the importance of having flexible attitudes toward activities that may indirectly influence how much meaning is experienced in a given occupation.

4. Occupation is the impetus that propels people forward.

In her Eleanor Clarke Slagle Lecture (Clark, 1993), Clark described the techniques of occupational storytelling and occupation storymaking. These therapeutic techniques are incorporated in an abbreviated and modified form in the Lifestyle Redesign Program; the reader is referred to other sources for a detailed discussion of this approach (Clark, 1993; Clark, Ennevor, & Richardson, 1996). Table 2 provides an overview of the key concepts.

In short, the approach begins with the therapist and client being open to discovering one another's perspective or standpoint on issues of relevance to aging and occupation. The goal is for each to become transformed by understanding a new perspective from the other. This process enables the therapist to gain insights into who

Table 2
Grounded Theory on the Technique of Occupational Storytelling and Occupational Story Making

Technique	Occupational Storytelling	Occupational Story Making

Collaboration	Evoke stories of occupation	Occupational coaching:
		    Encouraging positive remake
		    Offering occupational strategies
		    Reaffirming and marking progress

Building empathy	Analysis and synthesis:
	    Time
	    Value
		Evoking insight (problems and solutions)

Inclusion of ordinary		Broadened view of activities of daily living:
		    Handling emotion
		    Friendship and intimacy
		    Symbolic dimension of occupation

Listening		Image reconstruction
Reflection		Cultural place

the client is as an occupational being. The therapist next encourages the client to recount stories of his or her childhood along with adult occupations up to the time of the interview (occupational storytelling). Finally, the therapist and the client create a story that they will enact in the future, one that will promote the flourishing of the client as an occupational being.

In both the unabridged (described in Clark, 1993) and modified (used in the Lifestyle Redesign Program) versions of this approach, occupation is the impetus that propels people forward. In the process of occupational story making, the person decides on courses of action that he or she will enact in the next week or so. Experience, then, in the world of activity becomes transformational and generates new plans of action for the subsequent week. In this way, progressive growth, skill acquisition, and learning occur, and the sense of self is modified. In essence, life appears to be moving forward rather than stagnating.

Occupational storytelling and occupational story making capitalize on the recursive relationship between occupation and narrative (i.e., configuring the seemingly isolated episodes in one's life in terms of an unfolding and coherent plot) (Price-Lackey & Cashman, 1996). Through narrative, life events are made meaningful in the context of a forward-moving plot. One has the sense that one's life is unfolding with purpose and direction. Engagement in occupation, in turn, provides the kind of deeply felt experience that can reveal new aspects of the self to the participant. Experience in occupation can prompt one to revise his or her life story and self-image; however, how one is constructing the life history (or

story) will influence choices of occupation in the future. In the Lifestyle Redesign Program, we came to realize that, because of the recursive relationship between occupation and narrative, occupation served as the impetus that would move the participants forward to higher levels of challenge and accomplishment.

As a final note, although the general principles of occupational storytelling and occupational storymaking were adhered to in the Lifestyle Redesign Program, the abridged approach was modified for the group context. We found that, when stories were shared and enacted in a group context, this helped the participants to "stand back, gain perspective, and imagine new choices" (Belenky et al., 1997, p. 90) and to analyze more broadly the situations they thought were brought about by their personal ineptitude (Belenky et al., 1997). Furthermore, the group context for the doing and telling of stories created empathy and bonding among the participants.

Conclusion

In summary, the success of the Lifestyle Redesign Program resulted from helping the participants to acquire knowledge about the relationship between occupation and health and happiness, teaching them to use occupational self-analysis, encouraging the use of small steps in overcoming risk-taking fears, and promoting the use of skills gained in successful prior steps in an ongoing health-promoting daily routine. By using an incremental, additive approach, the participants developed new ways of viewing themselves and their potential to positively affect their future lives. ▪

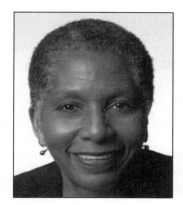

5

Content Modules

B elow is a list of themes that guided our treatment in the USC Well Elderly Study. The topics described are by no means exhaustive. They may spark new ideas and topics, and it is up to the therapist to decide how long to spend on any particular subject, depending on the emerging themes of each group.

- Occupation, health, and aging
- Transportation and occupation
- Finances and occupation
- Health through occupation: Physical and mental activity
- Dining as an occupation
- Time and occupation
- Home and community safety
- Relationships and occupation
- Outings, exploration, and special events
- Ending a group

We anticipated that each theme could be completed in approximately 1 month. However, each topic was used as a means of incorporating awareness of occupation and health within occupation. Because our groups had consistent members for 9 months, we discovered how important closure was for our closely bonded participants. We have included suggestions for making the ending of a Lifestyle Redesign Program group a time for celebration,

reflection, and positive transition. Please refer to Appendix 3 for sample handouts when applicable.

How To Use the Modules

As noted above, the modules lend themselves to flexible application. We have stressed that occupational therapy intervention should be pertinent for each person and every distinct group. This is what creates dynamic and meaningful outcomes.

Throughout group and individual interventions, the occupational therapist is continually aware of the goal toward occupational self-analysis. We integrated the concept of occupation within each module. For example, transportation was not just an isolated subject to discuss. We titled it "Transportation and Occupation" for the participants and addressed how the two were interrelated.

The first step in any group is to establish feelings of cohesion, safety, and rapport. This is formed through group rituals and roles. For example, participants can participate in setup and cleanup. One participant can write feedback on a large board while the other members initiate the ideas. Some participants can serve as mentors or assistants in basic group activities or when in the community on an outing.

To make the learning process more accessible to the participants in a Lifestyle Redesign Program group, the leader can modify handouts so that the print is large and easy to read. Handouts can be translated into another language if necessary. For some participants, handouts may not be as effective as discussion or demonstration. After the participants provide feedback on a subject, it may be helpful and affirming to create a handout with their responses. We discovered that the participants were delighted to see their feedback in print, and the handout validated their opinions as well as reinforced their memory.

We have included several tools to help you visualize, plan, and implement a Lifestyle Redesign Program. The first is a flow chart (Figure 5) that presents the steps in developing the program. Next, we have provided a sample schedule of themes and topics as one possible way to implement a program (Box 5). Finally, we include a planning sheet for organizing and designing each weekly session (Figure 6).

On the following pages are content modules. Within each module, we have included an introduction followed by potential group discussion questions and group activity ideas. Discussion questions and activities are meant to flow smoothly within a group. The occupational therapist can select ideas from each list and integrate them throughout a group session. Please refer to Appendix 3 for sample handouts described in the modules. ■

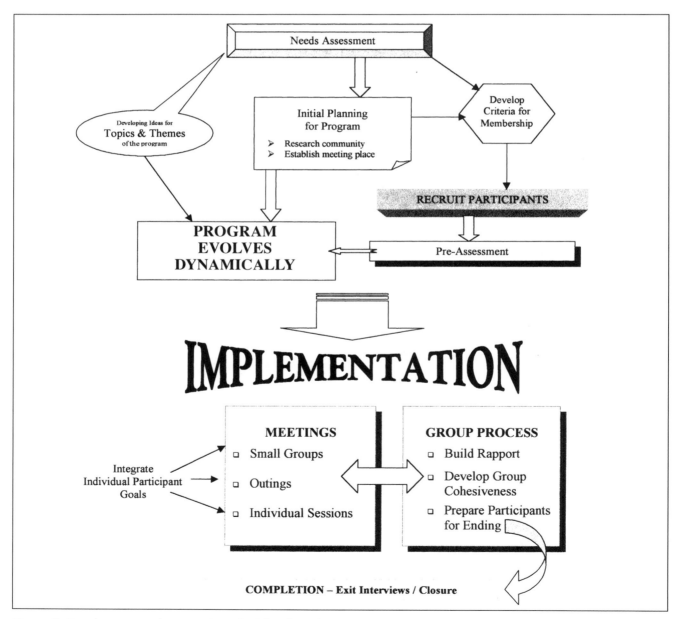

Figure 5. Development and progression of a Lifestyle Redesign Program.

Box 5
Sample Schedule for Implementing a Lifestyle Redesign Program

Week	Theme
1	Introduction to Occupation
2	Health and Aging: Changes in Occupation
3	Occupations: Time and energy
4	Outing: Healthy Occupation
5	Synthesis: Reflections on Occupation and Health
6	Transportation and Occupation: Introduction
7	Transportation and Occupation: Exploration of Resources
8	Outing: Bus Scavenger Hunt
9	Introduction to Stress Management
10	Stress Management Through an Active Body
11	Outing: Synthesize Active Body and Transportation
12	Occupations Requiring an Active Mind
13	Active Mind: Mental Challenges and Games
14	Outing to Library: Synthesis of Transportation, Mind, Body, and Stress
15	Introduction to Occupation and Dining
16	Nutrition: Guest Lecturer
17	Deciphering Food Labels
18	Adaptive Equipment in the Kitchen
19	Prepare for Cooking Group: Recipes and Adaptive Equipment
20	Cooking and Dining Together
21	Home Safety: Body Mechanics, Energy Conservation, and Fall Prevention
22	Adaptive Equipment in the Home and Joint Protection
23	Community Safety: Guest Lecturer From the Police Department
24	Safety Videos and Synthesis
25	Outing: Synthesis of Transportation, Healthy Occupation, Nutrition, and Safety
26	Healthy Pleasures Fair
27	Relationships: Personal Communication and Occupations as a Medium for Relationships
28	Cultural Awareness
29	Dealing With Loss
30	Outing: Cultural Exploration
31	Closure: Notebook and Review
32	Final Closure Outing
33	Closure: Notebook and Review
34	Graduation Party

Lifestyle Redesign Program

Date: _____   Week: _____   Theme: _____   Topic: _____

Occupational Concepts & Discussions Questions	Activities
1. Concept: Questions:	
2. Concept: Questions:	
3. Concept: Questions:	
4. Concept: Questions:	

Individual Goals:

Supplies:

1.
2.
3.
4.
5.

6.
7.
8.
9.
10.

Figure 6. Planning sheet for organizing and designing weekly sessions.

Occupation, Health, and Aging

The first step in a Lifestyle Redesign Program group is to clearly define what is meant by the word *occupation*. Many people define this term in a vocational context; however, we broaden the scope of meaning and apply it to the lives of elderly persons. Occupations are "chunks" of activity in which humans engage that can be named in the lexicon of our culture (Clark et al., 1991, p. 301). As occupational therapists, we can help elderly persons understand occupation in simple and practical terms.

For participants to begin to redesign their lifestyle, we offer them a critical tool so they may step back, reflect, and shape or reshape their thinking, thereby affecting their daily actions. In this module, the ultimate goal is to describe occupation in a new way (foundational occupational science concepts) and illuminate its relationship to health and to encourage elderly persons to apply this thinking in their own lives (occupational self-analysis).

Potential Group Discussion Questions

What Is Occupation?

How do people frequently define *occupation*?

Give examples of occupations in which you participate.

What occupations have you stopped participating during in the last couple of years?

What were your childhood occupations?

What are your present occupations?

During the last year, what new occupations have you tried that you have never engaged in before?

What have you always wanted to do? (This is a good lead question for outing preparation.)

The Aging Process and Occupation

How has the aging process affected your patterns of occupations?

How can positive adaptations enhance your occupations and quality of life?

How do you feel about aging?

What do you enjoy about getting older?

After viewing *The Sixth Sense* videotape (see Appendix 4) discuss the following:

- What obstacles do you face in your daily life?
- How would you like to change your environment (i.e., what would make the "perfect world")?
- What adaptations have you made to your home?
- What personal adaptations have you made in coping with the aging process?
- Do you experience ageism?
- How well do younger people understand the process of aging?

Personal Time, Energy, and Occupation

How do occupations shape our days (e.g., work, chores, meals, sleep and rest, clocks, and routines)?

What are your daily occupations?

When do you have the most energy to complete tasks?

What are your typical energy cycle patterns?

How would you fill the time if you had two more hours each day?

What has retirement meant for you? How was the transition process?

Discuss public versus private time.

How Is Occupation Related to Health?

What is health (e.g., physical, emotional, social, spiritual levels)?

What are your "healthy pleasures" (Ornstein & Sobel, 1989)?

What are your "unhealthy pleasures?"

After a community outing, discuss the following:

- In what ways did the outing promote health?
- How do occupations contribute to health?
- What other occupations promote health?

Group Activity Ideas

What Is Occupation?

Present slides on types of occupations (*Celebrating the familiar: The Sculptures of Seward Johnson, Jr.* [see Johnson {1987} in Appendix 4]).

Ask the seniors to record their present hobbies, projects, and daily occupations (*Daily Occupations and Hobbies* [handout in Appendix 3]).

Provide disposable cameras and ask group members to take pictures of themselves depicting their typical occupations to share with the group.

The Aging Process and Occupation

Discuss myths about aging (*What's Your Aging I.Q.?* [see handout in Appendix 3]).

Further discuss pertinent health issues (*Age Pages* [see the National Institute on Aging in Appendix 4]).

View T*he Sixth Sense* videotape (see Appendix 4), narrated by Arlene Francis, which addresses sensory changes related to aging.

Ask group members to share adaptive items or strategies they use around their home.

Personal Time, Energy, and Occupation

Create a group time line within a historical or cyclical framework (see the Time and Occupation module). Refer to *The Ageless Self: Sources of Meaning in Late Life* (Kaufman, 1986).

Recommended for individual intervention or advanced level groups:

- Ask the seniors how they organize occupations on a day-to-day basis (*Balance Your Life* [see handout in Appendix 3]).
- Encourage seniors, as appropriate, to keep a daily journal tracking their occupations.
- Challenge the seniors to go a day without wearing their watches.

How Is Occupation Related to Health?

Create your own *Words of Wisdom From Healthy Seniors: What Does It Mean To Be Healthy?* (see handout in Appendix 3) or make a list of healthy versus unhealthy occupations; determine which occupations contribute to the seniors' health during the morning, afternoon, and evening hours; or make a list of favorite health quotes or home remedies.

As a group, create a wellness mural that can be developed throughout the program or in one group session. Collect magazine clippings, pictures, phrases, and artistic interpretations of elderly persons involved in healthy occupations. You may want to include each participant's picture in the mural as well.

Share articles regarding health-producing occupations on such topics as humor, reminiscing, levels of stress, sensory input, leisure and other activities, and choice and personal responsibility.

Transportation and Occupation

We chose to introduce the topic of transportation and occupation early in our program. This offered the participants education and understanding before most of the outings into the community. The greater the preparation, the safer they felt in trying new steps and venturing out into the community. We strongly encouraged their participation because these outings provided the best opportunity for synthesis of the occupation-centered concepts they were learning.

The importance of the topic of transportation will vary according to the population with which you are working. For example, if most of the group members still drive their own cars, it is not as imperative to focus on public transportation. Public transportation is, however, an important issue for aging adults because many of them will eventually rely on public or special forms of transportation due to failing eyesight and physical or mental health problems.

There are several advantages to using public transportation for outings and exploration. First, public transportation can create group cohesion because participants share and learn new methods and resources available to them. These shared adventures create bonds. Second, public transportation can empower the group as they witness their ability to conquer unfamiliar territory. Third, as mentioned above, knowing multiple means of travel can be a tremendous resource for elderly persons to prepare for a time when they will use it extensively or for friends and family members who may likewise benefit from this resource.

We provide further information about transportation details in the Outings, Exploration, and Special Events module. It is critical that the therapist be well prepared for excursions, especially when relying on public and other organizations for safe and timely travel. This requires research and investigation on the part of the occupational therapist. However, often the best sources of firsthand information are the participants in the group.

Occupation is discussed in relation to each topic. For example, we challenged the participants to consider how transportation affects their occupations and vice versa. These core questions are listed first in the manual. However, in reality, they are to be integrated during the dynamic group interactions and throughout activity. The

therapist can create a pause for deeper reflection on the topic at any time, for example, by reminding the group of prior feedback they have given. Sometimes it is best to start with simple questions to lead into the "big picture." On other days, or with a different group, the therapist may determine that it is more effective to begin with the core occupational concept and follow up with more concrete examples. The key is to individualize intervention at all times and be ready to adapt the discussion while it is in progress.

Potential Group Discussion Questions

Transportation and Occupation

How does transportation affect your occupations? (*Sample Group Feedback: How Does Transportation Affect Occupation?* [see handout in Appendix 3]).

How do your occupations affect your transportation?

When is transportation itself an occupation?

When is transportation a means to an occupation?

Other Questions Related to Transportation

How have methods of transportation changed during your lifetime?

What types of transportation are available to you now?

What types of transportation do you use regularly?

What types of transportation are most economical (evaluate by cost, convenience, accessibility, aesthetic pleasure, etc.) (*Sample Community Transportation Resources* [see haṅdout in Appendix 3])

What types of transportation have you never tried?

How do transportation resources and constraints affect one's occupational choices?

What forms of transportation are available for people who use walkers or wheelchairs?

What reservations do you have about various means of travel?

Group Activity Ideas

Transportation and Occupation

Create a transportation resource information packet of services available to seniors living in a specific community that includes the following: telephone numbers, areas serviced, age or other requirements, wheelchair accessibility, cost, drawbacks, and helpful hints (see handout in Appendix 3).

Try out new methods of transportation together as a group such as community senior transportation services, public buses, subways, and trains (see the Outings, Exploration, and Special Events module).

Encourage seniors to sign up for their own bus pass, transportation service for elderly persons and those with disabilities, or other special services that are available in your community.

Provide brochures, maps, schedules, and telephone numbers whenever applicable.

Go on a scavenger hunt by bus where seniors are partnered up as teams to answer questions. This creates a greater awareness of their neighborhood within a fun and social context. Be sure to offer prizes. (*Community Exploration: Sample Bus Hunt* [see handout in Appendix 3]).

As a group, write a letter to the city's department of transportation to request the installation of a more convenient bus stop near the seniors' residence.

Encourage the seniors to participate as much as possible, and in many roles, for community outings. Facilitate the development of safe and more functional transportation skills.

Finances and Occupation

For many people, financial considerations constrain their choice of occupations. Seniors at most economic levels have an interest this issue, so it is helpful to use the topic of financial constraints for discussion and sharing. The way we use and view money is closely connected with our choices, values, and occupations. It is important to live within our financial limits without stifling our creative and novel participation in healthy occupations. We offer a word of caution, however, regarding the discussion of finances. The facilitator should be sensitive to cultural and personal differences that may encourage or discourage vulnerability in this area. Discussion should be free of competition, comparison, and even well-intended statements if those statements create a sense of inequality among group members.

Finances and Occupation is one of the most flexible modules. The level and manner in which it is addressed will vary according to location, site, and group participants. At Angelus Plaza, we anticipated that the participants would have modest incomes because of the housing requirements. We were prepared to provide education, facilitate discussion, and bring in guest speakers on topics such as Social Security, Medicare coverage, and money management. However, we discovered that these topics were well addressed by the facility. This meant we did not need to discuss financial matters at length. Instead, we scheduled the time to visit these lectures and attended the events as a group.

The theme of finance can be addressed briefly many times throughout a program as different themes are initiated. For example, the financial aspect is easily merged with the section on transportation and cost of travel. Or, as the group leader facilitates a discussion on dining, he or she may include cost-effective ideas along with the subject of nutrition and food labels. Education regarding financial choices can easily be included in the opportunities for synthesis offered by outings, exploration, and special events. Together, the group can choose inexpensive activities and means of travel as they share a healthy meal or exercise their mind and body when exploring a museum.

Potential Group Discussion Questions

How do finances affect your occupations?

How do occupations affect your finances?

Name something you would do, or a place you would go, if cost was not an issue?

How do you find meaningful occupations that are inexpensive? In other words, how can a senior stay healthy on a restricted budget?

Which restaurants, centers, activities, and markets are inexpensive or have discounts for seniors?

Which means of travel are affordable for you?

Where can you go to learn more about financial matters (e.g., Social Security)?

Define an occupation in terms of costs (e.g., financial, time, energy).

What is financial abuse, and how can you protect yourself from being a victim (see Home and Community Safety module)?

Group Activity Ideas

Have the seniors generate information from their own experiences and then create a booklet of inexpensive resources in their community (*Creating a Resource Booklet* [see handout in Appendix 3]).

Explore guides and resources for participation in inexpensive occupations. Bring in telephone books, newspapers, and so forth for a hands-on session on how to find cost-effective ideas in your neighborhood. Facilitate sharing among the seniors about senior discounts and opportunities (e.g., movies, museums, restaurants).

Create a packet of information regarding methods of available transportation and associated costs (see handout in Appendix 3).

Schedule a guest speaker on a topic pertinent to the seniors in your setting (e.g., a social worker, a Medicare provider representative, a financial abuse specialist).

Take an excursion to a free event or meeting (see Outings, Exploration, and Special Events module).

Health Through Occupation: Physical and Mental Activity

Healthy aging involves physical and mental stimulation. As the recently published MacArthur Study on Aging (Rowe & Kahn, 1998) indicated, much of the decline in mental and physical capacity associated with aging is explained by lifestyle factors rather than by genetics. In this module, participants learn that, if they do not regularly use their physical and mental capacities, they are more likely to lose them in the long term. The participants develop an appreciation that even the most seemingly mundane occupations, such as socializing with friends, knitting, or taking a short walk, can affect their health.

In the Occupation, Health, and Aging module, the participants discovered that health and well-being, as they relate to occupation, are determined by more than not being sick. Frequently, group members identified exercise as a healthy occupation. We spent time closely examining physical activity and, in addition, emphasized that exercising the mind is just as important as exercising the body. We included stress management and relaxation in this module to foster a balance between exercise and leisure. We found there to be an overlap between stress management and physical and mental health (i.e., breathing techniques and guided imagery), and these topics appeared to flow together well.

We emphasized a practical approach to incorporate these healthy occupations into participants' daily lives. They shared ways in which they were already integrating healthy occupations into their lives as well as easy ways to add more. For example, why not choose to take the stairs whenever possible instead of automatically pushing the elevator button? Participants became aware of how their mental and physical capacities were being stretched in activities they did every day such as the physical and cognitive aspects of preparing a meal.

Through our occupation-centered discussions, the participants became aware of many healthy occupations in which they were already engaged but had not realized until the USC Well Elderly Study. In addition, perspectives were reframed for some participants. For example, one gentleman thought that by relaxing he was being lazy. Through the group intervention, he was able to give himself permission to take time for relaxation.

We must offer a word of caution regarding intervention, especially when physical activity is introduced. We did not have access to the participants' medical information. If this information is not accessible to you, it is important that the therapist evaluate each participant's level of ability and judgment. The elderly persons in our program were independent adults and, for the most part, were able to communicate their limitations and needs. During individual sessions, the occupational therapist was able to discover more detailed information about a person's strengths and weaknesses. Even when all factors are known by participants and the therapist, it is always important to monitor and observe the responses of the participants and keep communication strong (e.g., during an exercise videotape, have participants learn to check their pulse and monitor any adverse symptoms).

Potential Group Discussion Questions

Stress Management and Relaxation

How is health related to relaxation?

How is health related to a balance of stress in our lives?

How do you keep your immune system healthy and active?

Take a look at the flow of your day and how you fill it (see Occupation, Health, and Aging module).

Share personal results from meditation or other stress-reducing activities such as attending church, gardening, or watching a sunset.

The Active Body: Physical Exercise

Why should we exercise?

What are the benefits of exercise?

What are different ways to be physically active?

How can you incorporate exercise into your daily life? (*Sample Group Feedback: How To Incorporate Exercise Into Daily Life* [see handout in Appendix 3])

How do you save your energy for valued occupations?

What is osteoporosis, and how can you affect bone density levels?

How do you deal with incontinence? [optional]

The Active Mind: Mental Exercise

Why should we exercise our minds?

What occupations exercise the mind?

What are some ways to improve memory? (*The Active Mind: Memory Tips* [see handout in Appendix 3])

Should memory be expected to fail with age?

What is the difference between typical forgetfulness and diseases of dementia?

Group Activity Ideas

Stress Management and Relaxation

View and participate in *The ROM Dance* (see Harlowe & Yu [1993b] in Appendix 4).

Rehearse relaxation techniques such as muscle relaxation, guided mental imagery, music and other sensory awareness, proper breathing, and massage.

The Active Body: Physical Exercise

View and participate in *The ROM Dance* (see Harlowe & Yu [1993b] in Appendix 4).

Learn to check your pulse rate as you exercise with the video *Living Younger Longer: Real People Getting Real Results* (1993 [see Appendix 4]).

Take a survey of the group members' level of activity (*How Active Is Your Body?* [see handout in Appendix 3]).

Take a tour of a senior center exercise gym and learn how to use the machines and weights safely.

Explore ways in which persons who use wheelchairs can remain active.

Incorporate exercise (e.g., walking, reaching, use of stairs) into an outing by adapting the physical level as needed for each senior.

The Active Mind: Mental Exercise

Share and play favorite board games, cards, and so forth.

As a mental challenge, put items on a tray, then take them away and see if the seniors can guess all of the objects.

Have one leader change clothes and accessories midway during a group session without letting the seniors know. See if they noticed and can remember what has changed.

Discuss myths about aging (see handout in Appendix 3).

Learn about an aspect of technology that is unfamiliar to participants (e.g., orientation to computers).

Dining as an Occupation

Cooking a meal together became a critical occupation for the Lifestyle Redesign Program groups. The process of creating a meal produced a social cohesiveness and helped unify the group members. For this reason, there is an argument for introducing the dining section earlier in the program. However, even if a cooking activity is introduced later on, it becomes a celebration of the growing relationships within the group.

The therapist should be aware that the group cooking activity usually requires more energy focused on preparation, setup, and cleanup than most other activities. Our program did not have access to cooking facilities (i.e., a kitchen) at our residential locations. Instead, we brought in our own burners, knives, cutting boards, bowls, coolers, and so forth.

The therapist should encourage the participants to be as involved as possible throughout the entire cooking group experience. This includes everything from planning the meal, to shopping together, to setup and cleanup. Some participants suggested bringing favorites dishes to share with the group. Once the meal was complete, group members made plates of food for those who were sick and absent that day and delivered them to their apartments.

By inviting a dietitian to speak to our groups before the cooking experience, we were able to incorporate healthy meal planning into the activity. The therapist took time to learn about the individual nutritional needs and concerns early to target this information through educational materials and discussion. We even sent the dietitian a list of pertinent questions, originating from group members, before her presentation.

We labeled our section Dining as an Occupation (versus Cooking or Nutrition) to emphasize the social and ritualistic aspect of meal sharing. It should be noted that, in an anthropological sense, dining is thought of as an occupation that has bonded tribes and communities throughout human history.

The themes of nutrition and food labels were steps toward cooking the meal and experiencing the ritual of dining. One group chose to dine in their activity center's cafeteria by making special arrangements with the kitchen staff members. We enjoyed a leisurely meal, complete with elaborate centerpiece and table, in a special dining area. The self-maintenance task of cooking and eating was transformed into a rich social and creative event.

It is important to note that the content on nutrition should not be handled in isolation but rather should be linked to the concept of occupation. For example, the participants must be aware that what we eat directly affects our energy levels and that an engaged life in the world of activity requires nutritional support at a different level than with a sedentary lifestyle.

Potential Group Discussion Questions

Dining and Occupation

What are your favorite foods?

How do eating and dining differ?

What are the differences between eating alone and eating with others? Which do you prefer? When and why?

What are all of the occupations leading up to and including dining?

Nutrition

(Questions directed toward a visiting dietitian)

What causes a high cholesterol level? What can you do to lower it?

How can nutrition or food help control high blood pressure?

Does cheese cause constipation?

How does a person determine what his or her healthy body weight should be?

How many times a day should a person eat (especially when trying to lose or gain weight)?

When cooking, which kinds of oil are the healthiest to use?

How effective are vitamins? What types should seniors use?

What are carbohydrates? How much of them do seniors need?

Understanding Food Labels

(Sample questions for *Food Label Quiz* [see handout in Appendix 3])

How many grams of saturated fat are in this item?

Which food contains more calories per serving?

What percentage of the Recommended Daily Allowance of sodium are in 5 crackers?

Other Topics

Homeopathic and herbal remedies

Medication and food interactions

Group Activity Ideas

Dining and Occupation

(After covering nutrition and food labels)

Use new information to plan and prepare a healthy meal together as a group.

Consider shopping as a group to integrate food label education.

Nutrition

Begin with a simple nutritional screening tool (*Determine Your Nutritional Health* [see handout in Appendix 3]).

Invite a dietitian to be a guest lecturer. This may be a good time to include information on medication interactions.

Follow up the lecture with a simple outline of material covered (*Sample Summary of a Nutrition and Medication Lecture* [see handout in Appendix 3]).

Take a kitchen safety quiz (*Can Your Kitchen Pass the Food Safety Test?* [see U.S. Food and Drug Administration in Appendix 4]).

Provide handouts from local health departments.

Take a shopping trip to the local farmer's market.

Create a group cookbook.

Understanding Food Labels

Answer questions and discuss the *Food Label Quiz and Definitions* (see handout in Appendix 3).

Review handouts such as *How To Read the New Food Label* (see handout in Appendix 3).

Other Topics

Test the group members' basic knowledge about medications (*Medications Quiz* [see handout in Appendix 3]).

Review *Medications: Things You Should Know* (see handout in Appendix 3).

Make sure that all participants have a list of their current medications in a secure location for physician visits and emergencies.

Time and Occupation

How people occupy their time is a core concept of occupational therapy. Few people, however, consciously reflect on this aspect of life, except for the fact that they never have enough time. By examining how our use of time affects us, we begin to see how to reshape or redesign our lives for a healthier outcome. This process helps elderly persons to appreciate more fully the way they organize and manage their time.

Life has tempo, which means it proceeds at a certain pace, and it is temporal, which means that, at any given moment, we experience the present in relation to our past and our future visions of ourselves (Clark, 1997). Typically, human beings have the sense that their lives are moving forward, but many elderly persons believe they are stuck or stagnating. In this module, we help the participants reflect on their lives in terms of its pace—past, present, and future—and in terms of forward progression. They learn about the experience of time and are encouraged to seize control of their time. They are given the sense that they can control time by virtue of what they do.

The theme of time is flexible in a program. It can be combined with other topics throughout the program and is discussed as Personal Time, Energy, and Occupation in the first section of the Occupation, Health, and Aging module. There may be situations where the occupational therapist deems it important to expand on the idea of time and how it relates to occupation.

A potential combination for the theme of time is with Dining as an Occupation. Discussion can be structured around holidays, celebration, and food. The following sections list potential questions and categorizes time as linear and cyclical.

Potential Group Discussion Questions

Linear Time and Occupation

(In conjunction with the historical time line activity)

What were the turning points, or milestones, in your life?

What makes an event or occupation a milestone in your opinion?

How are your milestones unique compared with the other group members?

How are we affected by historical events during our lifetime?

How are your decisions about occupations influenced by markers of time within a culture?

Cyclical Time and Occupation

(In conjunction with a pictorial display of seasons of the year)

Share a family ritual or tradition.

What are your daily, weekly, monthly, and annual patterns of occupation?

What events and holidays do you celebrate throughout the year?

How are events distinguished in other cultures?

How do these markers organize and affect our lives?

Group Activity Ideas

Linear Time and Occupation

Have each senior create their own time line depicting milestones and major events throughout his or her life.

As a group, illustrate a historical time line with personal overlay. Hang a large piece of butcher paper on the wall. Begin by filling in a historical time line (an almanac is helpful). Gradually add each group member's milestones or markers onto the same time line (start with birthdays).

During an individual session, create a Life History Video (see Appendix 2).

Cyclical Time and Occupation

On a large piece of paper or board, draw a circle and indicate seasons. By using group discussion, enter expected yearly events and holidays. Add each person's personal celebrations and markers to demonstrate unique qualities versus shared cultural rituals.

For more activities and handouts related to time, please refer to the Occupation, Health, and Aging module (see Personal Time, Energy, and Occupation section).

Home and Community Safety

Elderly persons are often in vulnerable circumstances due to physical or mental limitations, weakness, financial constraints, or isolation. Elderly persons are often targets for abuse and scams. For these reasons, many elderly persons refrain from engaging in occupation due to fear. We found that home and community safety was a topic all participants appreciate.

It is important to realize that elderly persons have established a lifetime of occupational patterns and habits, such as walking to a bank and cashing a welfare check at the same time and on the same day each month. Although it may be disruptive to change strongly embedded habits, we discussed how participants could make small changes that could prevent an unwanted attack.

Through the safety and consistency of the Lifestyle Redesign Program, we watched the participants find the freedom and courage to discover more options and healthier occupations. Novel occupations or once seemingly overwhelming obstacles became challenging adventures when tackled with a group led by a competent leader. The occupational therapist can gauge the level of activity for each member and provide teaching, coaching, and affirmation when needed. See the Outings, Exploration, and Special Events module for more tips on creating a safe environment for travel.

Finally, note that the topic of home and community safety is a sensitive matter. Please be aware that group participants may have been exposed to traumatic or violent events. At times, humor is a useful tool to lighten the mood. On the other hand, it is important for the therapist to acknowledge the gravity and consequences of this issue.

Potential Group Discussion Questions

Safety in the Home

Why is a safe environment important?

What are the major safety concerns in your life?

How does safety in the home affect your occupations?

Which occupations contribute to or hinder home safety?

What makes the home environment safe?

What are the common causes of falls?

Discuss disaster and emergency planning and preparation.

Safety in the Community

How might safety concerns inhibit occupations?

How might occupations enhance safety?

What keeps you from venturing into parts of your neighborhood?

How can seniors be safe in the community?

Personal Adaptations and Equipment

What adaptations have you made around your home to improve safety and efficiency?

Are any of your daily occupations potentially unsafe?

What activities would you consider changing or adapting to make them easier and safer?

How do you protect your body and joints from injury?

How do you conserve energy?

Group Activity Ideas

Safety in the Home

Complete a *Home Safety Evaluation* (see handout in Appendix 3) for each participant during an individual session. Have the seniors evaluate the safety of their homes by using a pictorial aid within a structured group session.

Set up emergency numbers and complete medication lists with each senior either in an individual or group session.

Rehearse safe risk taking, body mechanics, joint protection, and energy conservation techniques as well as fall prevention. The seniors in our program appreciated the opportunity to learn and practice how to get up from the floor safely.

Other recommended materials include

- *Safety Tips to Prevent Falls* (see handout in Appendix 3),
- *Home Safety Tips* (see handout in Appendix 3), and
- *The Do-Able Renewable Home: Making Your Home Fit Your Needs* (see Salmen [1991] in Appendix 4).

Safety in the Community

Review *Safety Outside the Home* (see handout in Appendix 3).

Ask the seniors to generate their own safety ideas and mottoes (*Group Feedback Ideas on Safety and Occupation* [see handout in Appendix 3]).

Invite a community police officer who is familiar with the neighborhood and crimes toward seniors to speak on such topics as community safety, elder abuse, financial abuse, and scams.

After the lecture, provide a clear and simple handout outlining highlights from the officer's presentation (*Sample Summary of a Police Safety Lecture* [see handout in Appendix 3]).

As an outing option, visit a local senior citizens center or library to hear a presentation on safety. For example, learn how to protect yourself from elder abuse, financial abuse, and scams.

Add creativity by role-playing safety scenarios. Ask the group members to identify ways to be as safe as possible. Please remember that this is a sensitive subject and should be handled carefully.

Personal Adaptations and Equipment

Present occupational therapy adaptive equipment and strategies, then explore and practice with adaptive equipment and techniques within an occupational context (e.g., a cooking group) or as a competitive game. For example, lift items with various reachers, use a magnifying sheet to read an article, open jars with a rubber grip, try one-handed techniques with adaptive equipment, or don a sock with a sock aid. If possible, distribute free items, such as pencil grip or jar opener, as well as sample equipment catalogs (refer to video summary *Arthritis and Everyday Living* [see handout in Appendix 3]).

Use an individual session to create a safe and efficient kitchen arrangement.

Borrow a wheelchair and allow the seniors to become familiar with this form of adaptation and to enhance awareness of disability.

Relationships and Occupation

Loneliness has been shown to notably compromise the health of elderly persons (Rowe & Kahn, 1998). One of the most crucial aspects of occupation that is health promoting is its ability to serve as a context for making and sustaining friendships. We have chosen to highlight community, communication, culture, and coping with loss as a major part of the content of this module. Each section can be developed further as indicated by the needs and desires of the group.

People often enter into social exchanges with little conscious thought about how relationships are formed. The focus on relationships creates an opportunity for reflection on the social aspect of the group as well as the meaning of relationships in each member's life. The occupational therapist can seize this opportunity to facilitate occupational self-analysis among the participants in the context of relationships.

As insight develops, the potential for greater understanding, growth, and change becomes possible. For example, after learning about the complexity of communication and recognizing the countless differences in people's perspectives and backgrounds, a group member may develop a greater tolerance for a neighbor who initially was perceived to be annoyingly odd. Furthermore, elderly persons learn specific ways in which occupation can be used as a way of promoting connectedness with others and avoiding social isolation.

Potential Group Discussion Questions

Relationships and Occupation

Describe your relationships with people in your life.

Why is community important?

How do social relationships affect occupations?

How can occupations be used to build relationships?

How do new relationships lead to new occupations?

Why does sharing our stories bring us closer together?

How does participation in an activity differ when you are alone versus when you are with other people?

How do you plan for an activity with other people?

In what ways does the aging process affect social relationships and community?

The Complexities of Communication

What obstacles have you encountered when planning an activity with other people?

What are helpful tips for effective communication?

Cultural Awareness

What is culture? How do we learn it?

Explore the concept of culture at various levels: national, urban, family, religious, and personal.

What is elevator etiquette, and how do we learn it?

How do we label persons of different ethnic origins?

What rituals and traditions are important to specific cultures?

How does culture affect occupation?

How do occupations affect culture?

How is culture infused into everyday occupations?

How can we be tolerant and understanding of differences in cultural styles?

Dealing With Loss and Grief

What feelings might a person experience after someone dies?

What do you do after you lose someone you love?

How do different cultures handle death and grief?

How can occupations be used to cope with the grieving process?

Group Activity Ideas

Relationships and Occupation

Think of places to go with people you know (*People–Places–Events* [see handout in Appendix 3]).

Take a closer look at the steps involved in planning activities (*Make a Plan* [see handout in Appendix 3]).

Plan events and outings together as a group.

Ask the seniors to document their social activities with photographs and share them with the group (e.g., provide them with disposable cameras).

During an individual session, create a Life History Video (see Appendix 2).

The Complexities of Communication

Introduce this section with a communication game (*Communication Building Blocks* [see handout in Appendix 3]).

Address aspects of physical appearance and presentation as a means of communication, including the following:

fashion, make up, manicure and nail care, body language, and posture.

As the seniors develop their own repertoire of resources, they may want to document and share them in a local or facility newsletter.

Cultural Awareness

Organize a heritage potluck luncheon where the seniors can share ethnic dishes.

Take a cross-cultural outing into the community (see Outings, Exploration, and Special Events module).

Explore children's games and occupations from participants' own backgrounds and cultures.

Dealing With Loss and Grief

Share resources, information, and support systems that are available to the seniors (Manning, 1984).

Outings, Exploration, and Special Events

Outings and special events provide opportunities to synthesize program concepts and principles through enactment. The seniors are able to practice and integrate health-promoting occupations into their lives. The experiences shared become a catalyst for further facilitation of their understanding of occupations (*Exploration as an Occupation: Sample Outing Memory Page for Notebooks* [see handout in Appendix 3]).

Exploring the community with a group of peers gave the seniors the chance to conquer their fears of novelty and change. The occupational therapist was always nearby to facilitate an appropriate level of challenge for individual group members. Each senior graduated from the Lifestyle Redesign Program with their own personal achievements and an improved sense of self-esteem and empowerment.

Finally, outings offered inherent health-promoting factors. Just being outside, actively engaging in activities of daily living, and focusing on community life increases one's quality of life. The occupational therapist capitalized on these experiences and used them as teaching tools. The group members were encouraged to build their willingness to take appropriate risks, develop friendships, and use available resources so that they would be more comfortable exploring the community without the coaching of the therapist.

Planning for Outings

The occupational therapist can encourage seniors to be actively involved in the decision making and planning of outings and facilitate member interactions and group independence. Before venturing into the community, the occupational therapist should do a trial run to foresee any problems. Anticipating obstacles and individual needs minimizes any fears the seniors have and promotes successful outings.

Initially, keep the plans simple and close to home. Over time, the seniors will develop more trust and rapport with the leader and other group members. Once they know they can succeed at smaller outings, they are generally more willing to participate in longer, more involved outings. Participants may even be comfortable accepting more of the responsibility for planning and implementing outings as their level of mastery increases.

Keep in mind the financial pressures that the seniors may be under. Learn together how to find cost-effective yet healthy and fun activities. With each outing, there are certainly group goals to which the therapist must attend (e.g., cohesiveness, social interaction, risk taking). On another level, each person on the outing has his or her own personal goals that can be incorporated (e.g., learning to mentor, strengthening muscles, improving balance and fine motor abilities, improving safety awareness and memory and independent problem solving).

Take the opportunity to stretch relationships and abilities in a more complex and less controlled environment. This tests a senior's abilities to maneuver in the community and emphasizes what the participant can do versus what the participant cannot do.

Details to Remember

Where are bathrooms along the way?

How often can we find shade?

Are there plenty of benches to sit on and rest as we travel?

How far is the walk from one bus stop to the next?

Are there elevators?

Make sure leaders have water, snacks, emergency kits, and contact information.

Potential Outing Sites

- Museum
- Library (an opportunity to explore computer technology and obtain a library card)
- Historical buildings
- Gardens
- Healthy restaurant
- Zoo
- Nearby city
- Cross-cultural neighborhood exploration (e.g., shopping, eating, touring)
- Volunteer for community events (e.g., cleanup, serving food, political action such as mailing letters or attending rallies for political causes)

- Craft fair
- Scavenger hunt on a bus route (see handout in Appendix 3)
- Nature hike
- Farmer's market
- Senior center gym and weight room
- Bank (an opportunity to learn how to use the automated teller machine)
- Focus on ecology and the environment by recycling or planting trees

Tours may be available at many locations.

Create Your Own Party

For more special occasions, celebrate with a party or fair. For example, we held a holiday gathering at Christmastime and, on another occasion, a heritage potluck luncheon celebrating cultural awareness. Encourage seniors to try new things, for example, to make a craft, try new foods, or learn how to line dance. Room decorations, music, and unique name tags can enhance the atmosphere. The seniors will have ample opportunity to be involved with planning, preparation, setup, and cleanup.

We created our own event, which we named "The Healthy Pleasures Fair." This fair was a way for our combined Lifestyle Redesign Program group members to experience the sense of well-being that comes from partaking of simple pleasures.

One large room was decorated with colorful streamers and balloons, transforming it into a place of festivity and celebration. As the seniors entered the music-filled room, they were directed to a table where they could design their own headpiece and receive a name tag. They were each given a "passport," a small booklet containing all of the possible occupations to explore that day. The passport hung around their necks by an attached cord so that their hands were free. At each station that they visited,

the corresponding page in the passport booklet was stamped. Later, this passport became a tangible reminder of all the new occupations they tried and the transformational effects of playful doing. It became a symbol of the adventure that they embarked on that day. Below is a list of the different Healthy Pleasures Fair station occupations.

- Games (ping pong, horseshoes, golf, darts, balloon volleyball)
- Computer games
- Pharmacist (checking your medications)
- Herbal tea tasting and healthy blended drinks (nonalcoholic)
- Guessing game (stereognosis activity)
- Massage
- Foot soak and podiatry evaluation
- Face painting
- Storytelling
- Crafts (picture frame, vase, or satin rose)
- Cookie decorating
- Gardening

The fair was presented to the participants as a celebration of small occupations that have the power to transform our lives. We could have simply told the seniors about the benefits of incorporating these activities into their lives, but the fair provided a medium in which they lost their sense of self, became immersed in pleasurable and engaging occupations, and ultimately experienced flow (Csikszentmihalyi, 1990).

The Healthy Pleasures Fair was a special event out of everyday time and place when a selected group of people shared a unique event. In this transformed time and place, seniors had the chance to experiment with new selves. The fair provided a multisensory context for play and exploration of occupation that primed the participants to open up to newness and change. The fair encouraged the Lifestyle Redesign Program group members to build images of who they have been, who they are, and who they can be through self-constructed occupation.

Ending a Group

The Well Elderly Group was different from other treatment settings. Traditional occupational therapy treatment is geared toward more individual intervention and often for a shorter time. Even when groups are activated, the members of those groups fluctuate from week to week as clients are able to participate and are admitted and discharged.

We tested groups that had fairly consistent membership for 9 months. There was a tremendous bond between group members and leaders as well as between the group members themselves. Telephone numbers were exchanged to facilitate interaction between participants outside of the group. One member told her group leader that she realized she had said something offensive toward another person in the group, so she initiated a call to her friend after the group ended to apologize.

It was difficult to let go of these relationships. The therapists and the seniors all felt a distinct sadness. Potentially, Lifestyle Redesign Program groups can be continuous; however, groups without a time limitation usually require additional members to maintain them over time, and this always affects dynamics. Again, there is great flexibility for occupational therapists in various settings to tailor the principles of the Lifestyle Redesign Program to their practice.

Below, we have provided ideas to help make the ending of a group a positive and hopeful transition. One aspect of saying goodbye is establishing meaningful rituals for each group and individual members.

Rituals for Closure

Begin preparations for the end of a group well in advance of the last meeting. The therapist can generate questions about transition and saying goodbye within group discussions. Allow the seniors a chance to express what the relationships have meant to them and how they have grown throughout the Lifestyle Redesign Program.

As the therapist nears the end of a Lifestyle Redesign Program, he or she can schedule group time to review content areas that have been covered previously. It is an excellent opportunity to integrate health issues with the participants' experiences of occupation. By now, the seniors have experienced many outings and therapeutic activities. At this point, the group members may be at a much deeper level of sharing and personal revelation because they have grown as a group and as individuals through the process of occupational self-analysis.

One way to structure the review process is through the Lifestyle Redesign Notebook. We helped the seniors put together their own Lifestyle Redesign Notebook as a means of reviewing program concepts and as a tangible way to remember the process they had experienced. We provided the seniors with a standard three-ring binder and labeled it with a creative cover unique to their group. Throughout the program, the seniors were encouraged to save their handouts; we ensured that they had a complete set of handouts by the end of the program. All of these handouts and exercises were assembled in sections behind a table of contents.

The seniors chose their favorite photographs, taken by the leaders throughout the program, and placed them in photo sleeves in their notebook. Permission to exchange telephone numbers was obtained so that we could provide a clearly typed list for each member. Members were encouraged to stay in touch with each other. Some groups enthusiastically planned to maintain their own social group independently once the therapist was no longer the designated leader.

We provided *Friends & Memories* handouts (see Appendix 3) for their notebooks with blank space for individual comments and signatures. We passed around each person's "Memory Page" and wrote comments of encouragement as if a school semester was ending.

The therapist typed a special letter for the group members, which was placed as an introduction for each notebook. Throughout the program, members brought in recipes, cartoons, poems, and other inspirational materials. The therapist made copies and included these contributions as well.

Finally, on the last day, the graduation ceremony took place. Seniors planned the day, which was made special by having a party complete with cake, decorations, and photographs. The seniors walked up to receive their certificates of completion to the tune of a graduation march. For some seniors, this was their first graduation ceremony. For all, it was a tremendously meaningful event and became a milestone marking their new awareness of health and occupation.

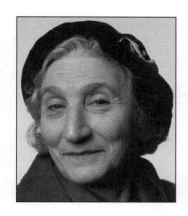

6

Outcomes and Reimbursement

The USC Well Elderly Study used five primary outcome measures (see Box 3 in chapter 1) to evaluate the effect of the occupational therapy intervention. Of these, the outcome measure that demonstrated the most dramatic results in the USC Well Elderly Study was the RAND 36-Item Health Status Survey, also known as the Short Form-36 (RAND SF-36; Hays, Sherbourne, & Mazel, 1993; Ware, Kosinski, & Keller, 1994; Ware & Sherbourne, 1992). This measure discriminates at higher levels of function more so than other assessments of function and was therefore appropriate for evaluating a group of independent-living older adults.

The reliability and validity of the RAND SF-36 has not been demonstrated for measuring outcomes of individual consumers. The Canadian Occupational Performance Measure (Law et al., 1994) is an appropriate alternative for measuring individual outcome for participants in a Lifestyle Redesign Program. A discussion of some of the features of each of these outcome measures follows. For a comprehensive overview of outcome measures, please refer to the American Occupational Therapy Association (AOTA) publication *Outcome Management and Program Evaluation Made Easy: A Tool Kit for Occupational Therapy Practitioners* (Forer, 1996).

The RAND SF-36

The RAND SF-36 is a self-report measure of health-related quality of life (HRQL) that was designed to measure health status efficiently from the consumer's perspective (Table 3). This instrument reflects a shift in the goals of medical care to preserve well-being and effective functioning of the consumer, and it is increasingly recognized that the consumer's experience of illness and treatment is required to achieve this goal (McHorney, Ware, & Raczek, 1993). Besides being a brief and efficient measure, one of the advantages of the RAND SF-36 is that it is a standardized (Stewart, Hays, & Ware, 1988) general health survey that can make comparisons across disease categories and health conditions.

The RAND SF-36 was developed as a subset of the larger (149 items) Medical Outcomes Study Questionnaire (MOS) (Hayes, Morris, Wolfe, & Morgan, 1995; Tarlov et al., 1989) that measures a person's general health and well-being. The MOS has been in use for nearly 10 years and has been shown to be valid and reliable across diverse groups, including older adults (Hayes et al., 1995); it is now being translated into many languages. The RAND SF-36 is a self-report survey that can be completed by the consumer in person or by mail or

Table 3
Sample Questions and Responses From the RAND SF-36

	Yes, limited a lot	Yes, a little	No, not at all
1. Does your health now limit you in			
• moderate activities such as moving a table, pushing a vacuum cleaner, bowling, or playing golf?	☐	☐	☐
• bending, kneeling, or stooping?	☐	☐	☐

	All of the time	Most of the time	A good bit of the time	Some of the time	A little of the time	None of the time
2. How much of the time during the past 4 weeks						
• did you have a lot of energy?	☐	☐	☐	☐	☐	☐
• have you been a very nervous person?	☐	☐	☐	☐	☐	☐
• did you feel tired?	☐	☐	☐	☐	☐	☐

administered as an interview. These features and the brevity of the RAND SF-36 make it an especially attractive tool.

The RAND SF-36 measures 8 domains (Table 4). Some of the health-related areas that are not covered by the RAND SF-36 but are addressed by more comprehensive measures like the MOS and the Sickness Impact Profile (SIP, 136 items; Bergner et al., 1981), include sexual functioning, sleep disorders, and family distress (Ware & Sherbourne, 1992).

The RAND SF-36 was designed for research and clinical applications. It has proved to be a valid and reliable measure of HRQL in research, especially for comparing groups, as was done in the USC Well Elderly Study. Its effectiveness is not as comprehensively documented at this time for cross-sectional and longitudinal research. Ware and Sherbourne (1992) indicated that the RAND SF-36 is sensitive for measuring HRQL for consumers with serious chronic diseases but suggested that, with a severely ill population, surveys be added that are more sensitive to the lowest end of the function continuum. (For a full discussion of the meaning of the various domains and the psychometric and clinical validity, see McHorney et al., [1993] and Ware and Sherbourne [1992]).

Use of the RAND SF-36 to measure clinical outcomes of individual patients should be approached thoughtfully. When the RAND SF-36 was used to evaluate large samples of patients receiving physical therapy

after three types of surgery, the nature of the surgeries resulted in different subscales being more or less sensitive (Mangione et al., 1997). Positive HRQL outcomes resulted a year or more after surgery when procedures had been more extensive, whereas other procedures had

Table 4
RAND SF-36 Domains

Domains	Number of items
General health	5
Mental health	5
Physical functioning	10
Social functioning	2
Role limitations attributable to physical health problems	4
Role limitations attributable to emotional problems	3
Bodily pain	2
Vitality	4

positive outcomes within 3 months. In other words, the types of procedures interacted with the timing of post-operative evaluation with the RAND SF-36 (Mangione et al., 1997). This example demonstrates how RAND SF-36 outcomes for a single person after, for example, 3 weeks of therapy, would not necessarily indicate whether the intervention was effective.

In addition to the ease of administration of the SF-36, it was a particularly appropriate measure to use in a population like that in the USC Well Elderly Study because it is sensitive to the levels of functioning found among independent-living older adults. Another measure of function, the Functional Status Questionnaire (Jette & Cleary, 1987), did not discriminate among variations in the higher levels of functioning among participants in the USC Well Elderly Study (i.e., it had a ceiling effect). However, a third instrument, the Life Satisfaction Z Index (Wood, Wylie, & Sheafor, 1969) was useful in detecting the effect of the Lifestyle Redesign Program on the subjective sense of well-being (Table 5).

Table 5
RAND SF-36 Advantages and Disadvantages

Advantages

- Self-report
- Brief
- General (not disorder specific)
- Multidimensional
- Well recognized
- Valid and reliable for some uses
- Measures functional abilities and effect on role performance

Disadvantages

- May not measure all domains of concern
- May have ceiling effects for high-functioning populations
- May have a floor effect for severely ill populations
- Usefulness in clinical applications is still being tested

Canadian Occupational Performance Measurement (COPM)

The COPM (Law et al., 1994) was developed to evaluate client-centered practice. It addresses function at the occupational performance area level and would therefore be appropriate for evaluating persons in an occupation-centered Lifestyle Redesign Program. The evaluation involves an occupational interview with the client that establishes problem areas that are defined jointly with the therapist. First, the client rates the importance of all identified problem areas on a scale from 1 to 10. The client additionally rates his or her ability to perform the identified activities and then his or her satisfaction with performance of the activity, also on a 1 to 10 scale.

The identified problem areas become the focus of occupational therapy goals and treatment, beginning with those areas rated by the client as most important. At reevaluation, performance and satisfaction scores are compared with beginning scores. The COPM measures the areas of self-care, productivity, and leisure and suggests activities for these areas but encourages practitioners to use these activities only as a guide. Therefore, the COPM is highly individualized to the specifics of a client's life, needs, and values. The COPM currently has not been validated as a true measure of change of occupational performance. Some of the advantages of the COPM are that it directly addresses occupational performance and provides a numerical value that can easily be used in analyses. For complete information on the COPM, contact the Canadian Association of Occupational Therapists, Toronto, Ontario, Canada for the test manual, or attend an AOTA workshop on the COPM (Table 6).

Goal Attainment Scale (GAS)

The GAS (Ottenbacher & Cusick, 1990) provides a means of standardizing change scores that result from occupational therapy treatment so that change can be compared across various disorders and differing treatments. The GAS consists of "five non-overlapping levels of concrete observable goal behaviors" (Trombly, Vining, & Radomski, 1998, p. 812) that increase in function at each level. These behaviors relate to a goal that has been collaboratively established by the client and

Table 6
COPM Advantages and Disadvantages

Advantages

- Client perspective guides process

- Directly measures occupation

- Addresses client specifically

- Demands practitioner–client collaboration

- Quantifiable results

Disadvantages

- Not a validated measure

- Numerical values may not represent the equivalent degree of change in ability or satisfaction when outcomes of two or more clients are compared

practitioner. The levels are coded as –2, –1, 0, +1, and +2, with the –1 level reflecting the client's level of function at the beginning of treatment. The 0 level indicates the level of behavior that is expected at discharge. This method has been found to be valid and reliable as an evaluation of occupational therapy interventions (Malec, Smigielski, & DePompolo, 1991).

Trombly and associates (1998) combined the COPM and GAS methods to evaluate achievement of self-identified goals in adults with traumatic brain injury. The COPM was used to identify occupational performance areas of functioning about which the participants were concerned. Participants completed the process of rating these areas for importance, ability, and satisfaction at intake, at discharge, and at follow-up. The areas of performance deficit became the basis for establishing appropriate and relevant goal attainment scales. The GAS scores made it possible to compare a client's performance before and after treatment and will make it possible to compare one client with another (Table 7).

Summary

The RAND SF-36 is a widely recognized measure of HRQL, a measure that is increasingly included when the effect of medical and treatment protocols is evaluated. Patient self-ratings of function and overall well-being are reliable and central to evaluating the experience of illness, rehabilitation, or meeting the challenges of everyday life such as with the participants in the USC Well Elderly Study. However, the RAND SF-36 is not a "magic bullet" outcome measure for occupational therapy interventions. It was particularly well suited to evaluate the population in the USC Well Elderly Study. Many of these older adults experienced functional deficits at an occupational performance level but were independent in basic activities of daily living (Clark et al., 1997), and all lived independently, although some had support services. The RAND SF-36 is an important instrument that must be added to the occupational therapy repertoire. The COPM, GAS, and Life Satisfaction Z Index are potential alternatives for measuring outcomes of the Lifestyle Redesign Program in clinical settings.

Reimbursement

In 1995, 33 million people (nearly 13% of the U.S. population) were 65 years of age or older (U.S. Bureau of the Census, 1996). Projections suggest that, by the year 2020, this segment will grow to 17% of the population, and of this group, more than 40% will be more than 75 years of age (U.S. Bureau of the Census, 1992). More

Table 7
Goal Attainment Scale Advantages and Disadvantages

Advantages

- It measures change that is specific to occupational therapy interventions

- Standardized score allows comparison of client outcomes

Disadvantages

- Creating 5 clear, concrete, observable, related behaviors for each problem is difficult

- The absolute increase in function between levels may vary rather than the even distribution suggested by the –1, 0, +1 scaling

- The actual increase in client function represented by one level may vary between one practitioner and another

people are living longer every year but are not necessarily living quality lives. Many elderly persons are living with chronic disabilities, and studies indicate that this trend is not abating (Crimmins, Haywood, & Saito, 1994). The first and best strategy to deal with this issue is prevention.

The USC Well Elderly Study has demonstrated that a program of lifestyle redesign can improve quality of life or slow the declines in health and maintain independence for elderly persons (Clark et al., 1997). This study coincided with a growing movement to understand and promote successful aging (e.g., Carlson, Clark, & Young, 1998; Ory & Cox, 1994; Rowe & Kahn, 1998). More retirement communities are developing wellness programs and fitness centers. Managed care facilities are promoting prevention and wellness because they realize that keeping people healthy costs less than long-term nursing care. Occupational therapy and Lifestyle Redesign Programs are a timely response to this growing need.

The USC Well Elderly Study is the best tool a practitioner can use when he or she is beginning the process of acquiring funding for a Lifestyle Redesign Program. This study not only demonstrated the effectiveness of the program, but also it showed that the results are sustainable and cost effective (Clark et al., in press). Because of its cost effectiveness, the Lifestyle Redesign Program is a program in which practitioners can engage in occupation-centered practice and maintain humanistic values (Burke & Cassidy, 1991).

Reimbursement Suggestions and Strategies

- Managed care systems set aside money for health edu-cation and wellness. Seek funding from these sources rather than from treatment sources.
- Seek public and private grants to fund lifestyle redesign programs in community settings.
- Private clients who can afford to do so may want to fund an individualized program for lifestyle redesign to meet their needs specifically.
- Rearrange current individualized treatments into group treatments to use adapted lifestyle redesign methods.
- Two important guidelines that recommend coverage by Medicare Part B for occupational therapy services are currently being drafted. These guidelines support reimbursement for adapted versions of lifestyle redesign, and include guidelines for functional maintenance programs whereby a physician could order therapies for the recovery of activities of daily living skills, and guidelines for rehabilitation services delivered in group settings for up to four persons where individualized goals are met as well as group goals.
- Talk about the USC Well Elderly Study to colleagues and administrators and they may decide to reallocate current funds, remember the study when new funds become available, and support efforts to locate funding.

Since the publication of the results of the USC Well Elderly Study, the investigators have received hundreds of requests for more information about the Lifestyle Redesign Program and requests to duplicate the research study. Interest has been expressed by occupational therapy practitioners, physical therapists, and physicians. The reader is encouraged to promote the USC Well Elderly Study because professionals are eager to hear about it. ■

Appendix 1
Individual Sessions

The Lifestyle Redesign Program was designed to draw strength from one-on-one interactions as well as from weekly group sessions. Groups provide opportunities to educate, develop rapport, and gain information about what is important or needed for participants and to facilitate social interaction.

Individual treatment times are an opportunity to discover, plan, and implement a personalized program of lifestyle redesign. In these sessions, occupations that would enhance the participants' health and well-being can be added, reintroduced, or facilitated by creating a customized plan of meaningful occupation that will carry over after the program's end because it will be anchored in the participant's daily routine.

Included below are topics that would be appropriate for individual sessions in a lifestyle redesign program.

- Develop an individualized (customized) plan of lifestyle redesign.
- Evaluate the participant's sense of place and note meaningful objects in the environment.
- Reinforce group session content. Bring a participant up to date on a session he or she missed. Work with a person who wants to explore a topic area in greater depth.
- Provide traditional occupational therapy intervention as needed. Provide home safety and risk evaluation. Address traditional occupational therapy issues if the scope is limited.

If more than two sessions are needed, refer the participant to additional occupational therapy or an appropriate professional.

Appendix 2
Life History Video

The Lifestyle Redesign Program incorporates occupational storytelling and occupational storymaking as described by Clark, Ennevor, & Richardson (1996). As part of this process, the participant provides a history of his or her occupations from childhood through the present. He or she is assisted in developing a vision of a future he or she desires. As part of this process, participants were encouraged to produce a videotape of their history as an occupational being.

Below, we have included some suggestions for initiating the Life History Video. All of these strategies are broad and tend to be conceptual—they are only a "door." Once the door is open, use a comment to guide the interviewee to the specific, such as, "Tell me about ..." or "What was your bedroom like?"

- Tell stories.
- Paint or draw a picture.
- Describe the setting.
- Tell me about that.
- Use a photo album to elicit stories.

The following are some additional questions to begin the life history process.

- If your life is a book, what would you name the chapters?
- What are three pieces of wisdom, or messages, from your life that you want to share [themes of meaning]?
- What are three events that you believe were important in shaping you and your life?
- How do you see yourself (humanitarian, good person, artist, etc.)? What are four ways you identify yourself?

Presenting the Life Video Process

We found the following logistics worked well when preparing participants for this project.

- Introduce the video concept during a group session.
- Ask participants to spend some time thinking about why they want to participate and what they want to discuss.
- Set up an individual session.
- Select backup questions from the list provided.
- In an individual 2-hr or more session, tape the video; practice what they want to cover, then tape the video; or tape a practice video.
- The completion of this process may take several individual sessions.

Appendix 3
Module Handouts

The Active Mind: Memory Tips

Arthritis and Everyday Living

Balance Your Life

Communication Building Blocks

Community Exploration: Sample Bus Hunt

Creating a Resource Booklet

Daily Occupations and Hobbies

Determine Your Nutritional Health Checklist

Exploration as an Occupation:
Sample Outing Memory Page for Notebooks

Food Label Quiz

Food Label Quiz and Definitions

Friends & Memories

Group Feedback Ideas on Safety and Occupation

Home Safety Evaluation

Home Safety Tips

How Active Is Your Body?

How To Read the New Food Label

Make a Plan

Medications: Things You Should Know

Medications Quiz

People–Places–Events

Safety Outside the Home

Safety Tips To Prevent Falls

Sample Community Transportation Resources

Sample Group Feedback:
How Does Transportation Affect Occupation?

Sample Group Feedback:
How To Incorporate Exercise Into Daily Life

Sample Summary of a Nutrition and Medication Lecture

Sample Summary of a Police Safety Lecture

What's Your Aging I.Q.?

Words of Wisdom From Healthy Seniors:
What Does It Mean To Be Healthy?

The Active Mind: Memory Tips

1. Be organized. Put everything in a specific place.

2. Write notes for yourself and make lists.

3. Use a calendar or appointment book.

4. Post reminders on doors, the refrigerator, or a mirror.

5. Use a timer or whistling kettle.

6. Immediately file important papers.

7. Re-check papers or double-check trash if necessary.

8. Use word or letter associations.

9. Retrace your steps to jog your memory.

10. Use a routine to your advantage.

11. Don't rush. Pause and be patient; you may remember.

12. Be prepared with emergency numbers and kit.

13. Keep your mind sharp. Use it or lose it!

14. Remember that everyone, no matter what age, has moments of forgetfulness.

Arthritis and Everyday Living

Always use good posture when performing any activity.

Whenever possible, sit rather than stand (keeping hips, knees, and ankles at a 90 degree angle). Frequently change positions.

Try sliding instead of lifting objects.

If you must lift, use good body mechanics:
- Bend at the knees
- Pick up object with both hands
- Use the larger muscle groups

Carry objects close to your body.

Prioritize the order in which chores have to be done.

Perform work at a moderate pace.

Alternate between light and heavy chores.

Reduce the number of trips to particular areas.

Store most used items in easily accessible areas.

Use lightweight equipment.

Avoid overly stressful activities, which can cause joint damage.

Don't overdo it. Pace yourself, scheduling regular rest intervals in order to increase endurance. Even five to ten minutes of rest during an activity can reduce pain and stress.

Information from the video "Arthritis and Everyday Living"
A/V Health Services, Inc. P.O. Box 20271, Roanoke, VA 24018

BALANCE

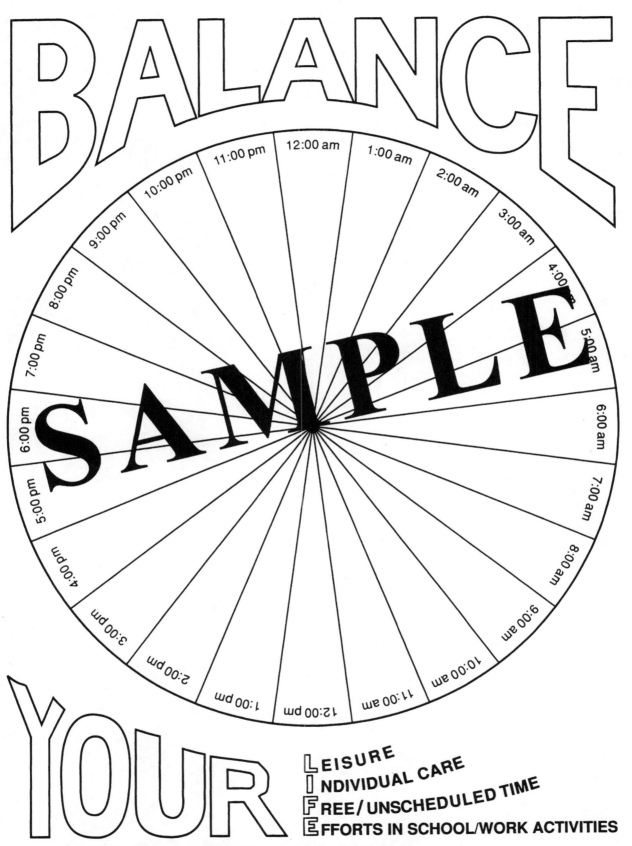

YOUR

LEISURE
INDIVIDUAL CARE
FREE / UNSCHEDULED TIME
EFFORTS IN SCHOOL/WORK ACTIVITIES

COMMUNICATION BUILDING BLOCKS

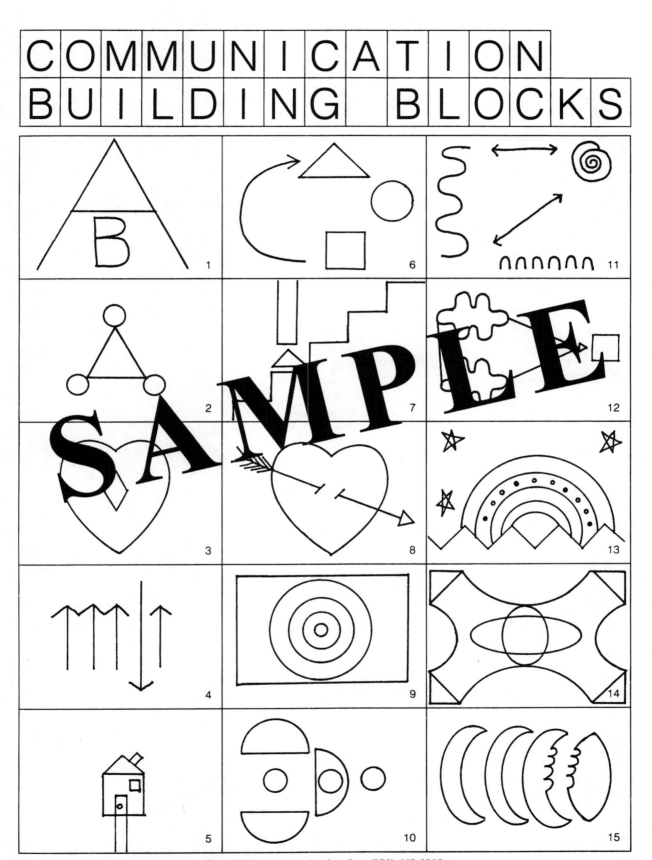

Community Exploration
Sample Bus Hunt

1. The Post Office is at the corner of Colorado Blvd. and _____.

2. What is the name of a restaurant on Colorado Blvd.? _____

3. We are traveling along Historic Route Number _____.

4. Thieves Market sells what kind of product? _____

5. When is the Norton Simon Museum open? _____

6. How far west does the bus go on Colorado Blvd.?
   Name the street: _____

7. The color of the Green Hotel Apartments is really _____.

8. Name a bank on Green Street: _____

9. What is playing at the Pasadena Civic Center? _____

10. Is this bus wheelchair accessible? _____

11. What color are the roses at Del Mar Ave. and Lake Ave.?
    (Look to the right): _____

12. What is your favorite restaurant on Lake Ave.? _____

13. Name a movie playing at the Academy Theatre: _____

14. You can make Xerox copies at _____.

Get off the bus after Oakland Ave. for more city exploration and fun!

Creating a Resource Booklet

The participants in a Lifestyle Redesign Program can create their own resource booklet. This is a personalized guide containing information about the neighborhood community and all that it has to offer seniors. The following is a list of potential categories to cover in your resource booklet.

- **Transportation Options**
  Such as buses, vans, and subways

- **Entertainment Ideas**
  Such as concerts, market places, hospital fairs, and special tours

- **Museums**

- **Food**
  Such as restaurants and places where senior discounts are offered

- **Household Items and Services**
  Such as free legal services

- **Things To Do That Are Free**
  Such as library activities, poetry reading, or playing cards with friends

It may be helpful to include prices, senior discounts, and contact numbers for events. Depending on the members of your Lifestyle Redesign Group, the booklet can include only inexpensive ideas or more expensive options as well.

To foster independence among the elderly, we included a page in our booklet describing where to learn about other events and ideas. The seniors were instructed to look in papers (i.e., residence newsletters, newspapers, phone books, city publications) and to watch for information posted on bulletin boards and in flyers around their community. We encouraged them to ask questions in their community such as when happy hours, specials, and discounts are available at restaurants.

Daily Occupations and Hobbies

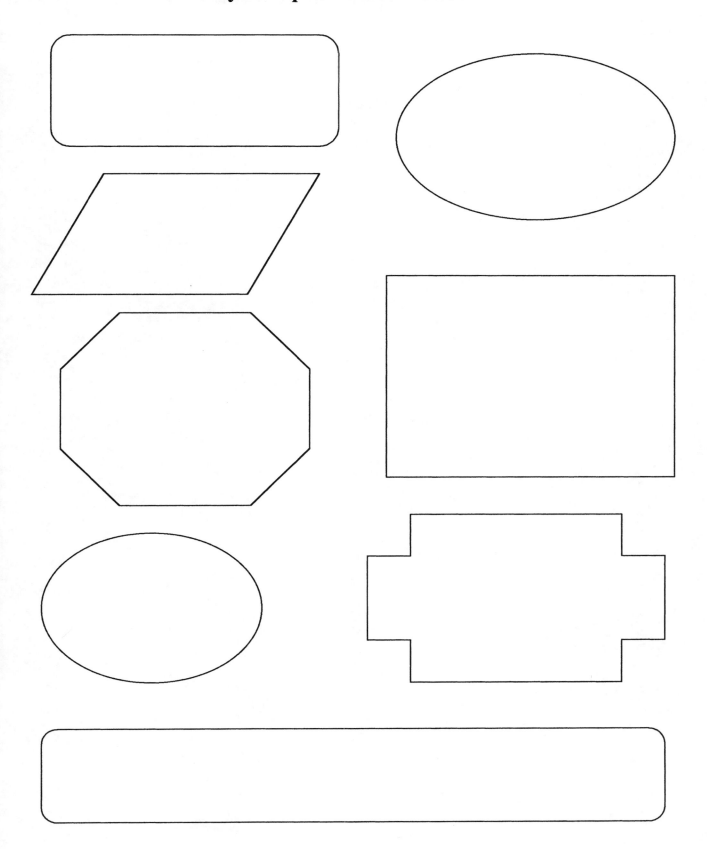

Determine Your Nutritional Health Checklist

Read the statements below. Circle the number in the yes column for those that apply to you or someone you know. For each yes answer, score the number in the box. Total your nutritional score. To interpret your score, consult the American Academy of Family Physicians web site at *www.aafp.org/nsi/e-determ.html.*

I have an illness or condition that made me change the kind and/or amount of food I eat.	◯ Yes (2 pts.)
I eat fewer than 2 meals per day.	◯ Yes (3 pts.)
I eat few fruits or vegetables, or milk products.	◯ Yes (2 pts.)
I have 3 or more drinks of beer, liquor or wine almost every day.	◯ Yes (2 pts.)
I have tooth or mouth problems that make it hard for me to eat.	◯ Yes (2 pts.)
I don't always have enough money to buy the food I need.	◯ Yes (4 pts.)
I eat alone most of the time.	◯ Yes (1 pts.)
I take 3 or more different prescribed or over-the-counter . drugs a day	◯ Yes (1 pts.)
Without wanting to, I have lost or gained 10 pounds in the last 6 months.	◯ Yes (2 pts.)
I am not always physically able to shop, cook and/or feed myself.	◯ Yes (2 pts.)

Reprinted with permission by the Nutrition Screening Initiative, a project of the American Academy of Family Physicians, the American Diabetic Association, and the National Council on the Aging, Inc. Funded in part by a grant from Ross Products Division, Abbott Laboratories.

Exploration as an Occupation
Sample Outing Memory Page for Notebooks

The Bradbury Building: *Exploring the neighborhood*
                             Physical exercise
                             A sense of history

This building is a historical landmark built in 1893 in downtown Los Angeles. We tried the old-fashioned elevator, visited a politician, and walked down all five flights of stairs, exploring as we went.

Los Angeles Central Library: *Learning from one another*
                                   Challenging our minds

Mimi paved the way by foot over to the library where our wonderful tour guide amazed us with facts about the incredible building.

Baja Mexican Grill Restaurant: *Healthy dining*
                                     Trying new food and drink
                                     Adapting transportation methods

Rain or shine, we enjoyed inexpensive, fresh food in Pasadena. Some took dial-a-ride, others a taxi, but we all got to taste healthy juice drinks with our lunch.

Los Angeles Zoo: *Playful environment*
                       Physical endurance
                       Traveling in style

We survived the trip to the zoo via a decorated Pasadena free bus. Some came for the food, others for the gorillas. Maggie said she just wanted to visit her relatives! Bravo to those who made it with canes or wheelchairs and to those who pushed those chairs.

Food Label Quiz
To be used with sample food products and packages

1. Rate cooking oils in order from the most healthy to the least healthy:

   _____
   _____
   _____
   _____

2. How many grams of dietary fiber would you get from a one cup serving of:

   Grape Nuts?   _____
   Cheerios?   _____
   Rice Chex?   _____

3. Is the fruit punch, snapple drink, or diet coke healthier? Why?

   _____
   _____
   _____

4. What are the three main differences between the chunk light tuna and the solid white tuna?

   _____
   _____
   _____

5. Which brand of breadcrumb is best if you are on a low salt diet?

   _____

6. List these snack foods in order from most to least healthy:

   _____
   _____
   _____
   _____

Food Label Quiz and Definitions

1. **Net weight** means: a) weight of contents
                                    b) weight of package
                                    c) weight of package and contents

2. **Nutrition information** on a food product label gives facts about:

                                    a) weight and price
                                    b) how to serve
                                    c) how the body uses the food

3. **Ingredients** means: a) cautions
                                    b) contents
                                    c) dosage

4. A **perishable** food means one that: a) contains many calories
                                                b) has no artificial ingredients
                                                c) spoils easily outside a refrigerator

Definitions

Net weight: weight of what is inside the package

Nutrition: the way the body takes in and uses food

Ingredients: what a product is made of or contains

Perishable: spoils easily

Calories: units of food energy (When you eat more calories than you need, you gain weight.)

Gram: approximately the weight of a paper clip (measurement in the metric system)

Friends & Memories

Group Feedback Ideas on
Safety and Occupation

Group One: Think safety both **in** and **outside** the home (for example as you plan, cook, groom, housekeep, and visit friends)

Group Two: During your daily life, as your mind is busy, ask yourself if you are still aware of your surroundings. **Balance** safety with activity; this means not rushing around too fast.

Group Three: Make your home efficient for activities yet safe, with minimal clutter. Try not to buy things that you don't need, only the things that you need to keep safe.

Group Four: A safe environment leads to a better lifestyle, extended lifespan, and better health and habits. These, in turn, lead to a **quality of life** of activity and happiness.

Home Safety Evaluation

Name:
Address:

Safety hazards will be circled below.

Comments:

Entrance & Exit
- Able to open door
- Able to use key
- Able to open sliding door, locks, windows

Living Area
- Scatter rugs
- Electric and phone cords
- No sharp, protruding furniture
- Couch or chair firm and high; support neck and back
- Ample, no-glare lighting
- Room temperature

Kitchen & Dining Room
- Rugs and mats
- Able to use faucets with ease
- Safe use of oven, stove, and microwave
- Arranged for accessibility and safety
- Appropriate seating height at table

Bedroom
- High and firm bed and mattress
- Positioning during sleep
- Access to light switch or lamp

Safety hazards will be circled below.

Comments:

Bathroom
- Rugs and mats
- Able to use faucets with ease
- High enough toilet seat
- Grab bars accessible
- Grab bars securely attached
- Tub and floor mats
- Able to reach emergency cord from floor

Additional Equipment:

Other Emergency Precautions
- Telephone locations
- Emergency numbers on phones
- Ringer and dial tone loud enough
- Functional smoke detectors
- Updated medical information easily accessible
- Earthquake and emergency preparations made

Further Comments:

Date:
Evaluation Completed by:

Home Safety Tips

Bathroom

- Grab bars should be securely attached to wall supports.
- The tub, shower, and bathroom floor should have a nonskid surface.
- A safe bath chair or bench helps to conserve energy and compensates for balance or strength problems.
- Raised toilet seats make it easier to sit down and rise up.

Telephone

- Emergency numbers should be available on or beside each phone and easy to read. Adapted push button covers can be placed over the phone with enlarged numbers.

Kitchen

- Use step stools that are safe and stable, with an extension that supports balance.
- Frequently used items should be stored within reach.
- Dials on the stove, oven, and microwave should be large enough to read with ease.

Living Room

- Furniture should be arranged to allow a clear path for walking.
- Low pile carpets are safer than think pile carpets.
- Scatter rugs should have nonskid backing.
- Extension and other cords should be clear of walkways and should not be under furniture legs or carpet.

Assistive Devices

- Key holders, jar openers, adapted scissors, doorknob turners, etc. can help increase function and comfort.

How Active is Your Body?

Name: _____
Date: _____

1. What activities or sports did you participate in when you were younger?

2. What is your favorite physical activity now?

3. If you exercise, how often do you do it?

4. What kind of physical activity do you participate in currently?

5. What, if anything, limits your participation in physical activity?

6. Would you like to exercise more?

What's Good About the Label?

It's simple. Healthy eating has never been easier, thanks to the nutrition label. Here are the facts:

- Most foods in the grocery store must have a nutrition label and an ingredient list.

- You can buy with confidence. Claims like "low cholesterol" and "fat free" can be used only if a food meets legal standards set by the government.

The nutrition label is titled *Nutrition Facts.*

Why Read the Label?

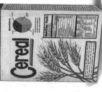

Read the label to help choose foods that make up a healthful diet. Eating a healthful diet can help reduce your risk factors for some diseases. For example, too much saturated fat and cholesterol can raise blood cholesterol (a risk factor for heart disease). Too much sodium may be linked to high blood pressure. High blood pressure is a risk factor for heart attack and stroke.

No one food can make you healthy. In addition to eating healthful foods, stay active, don't smoke, and watch your weight!

How To Read The Food Label

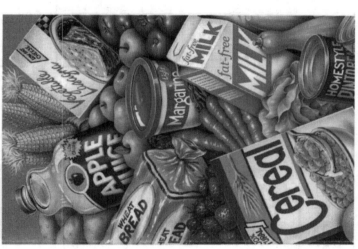

The guidelines in this brochure are for healthy adults and children aged 2 or older. A low-fat diet may be harmful to children younger than 2. For information on special diets, contact your physician or a Registered Dietitian (R.D.) or a Licensed Nutritionist.

For more information on nutrition, heart health and disease, contact your nearest American Heart Association or call 1-800-AHA-USA1 (1-800-242-8721), or online at www.americanheart.org.

Text and graphics are in the public domain and may be reproduced without permission.

You Can Rely on the Food Label

Rest assured, when you see key words and health claims on product labels, they mean what they say as defined by the government. For example:

Key Words	What They Mean
Fat Free	Less than 0.5 gram of fat per serving
Low Fat	3 grams of fat (or less) per serving
Lean	Less than 10 grams of fat, 4.5 grams of saturated fat and no more than 95 milligrams of cholesterol per serving
Light (Lite)	⅓ less calories or no more than ½ the fat of the higher-calorie, higher-fat version; or no more than ½ the sodium of the higher-sodium version
Cholesterol Free	Less than 2 milligrams of cholesterol and 2 grams (or less) of saturated fat per serving

To Make Health Claims About...	The Food Must Be...
Heart Disease and Fats	Low in fat, saturated fat and cholesterol
Blood Pressure and Sodium	Low in sodium
Heart Disease and Fruits, Vegetables Grain Products	Low in fat, saturated fat and cholesterol, and contain at least 0.6 gram soluble fiber, without fortification, per serving
Heart Disease and Soluble Fiber (such as foods containing whole oats or psyllium)	Low in fat, saturated fat and cholesterol, and contain at least 0.75 gram soluble fiber per serving from whole oats or 1.7 g soluble fiber from psyllium husk.

Other claims may appear on some labels.

Total Fat

Aim low: Most people need to cut back on fat! Too much fat may contribute to heart disease and cancer. Try to limit your **calories from fat**. For a healthy heart, choose foods with a big difference between the total number of calories and the number of calories from fat.

Saturated Fat

A new kind of fat? No — saturated fat is part of the total fat in food. It is listed separately because it's the key player in raising blood cholesterol and your risk of heart disease. Eat less!

Cholesterol

Too much cholesterol — a second cousin to fat — can lead to heart disease. Challenge yourself to eat less than 300 mg each day.

Sodium

You call it "salt," the label calls it "sodium." Either way, it may add up to high blood pressure in some people. So, keep your sodium intake low — less than 2,400 mg each day (100% Daily Value).

Daily Value

Feel like you're drowning in numbers? Let the Daily Value (DV) be your guide. A food with 5% DV or less has a small amount of the nutrient; 20% DV or more is a lot. For fat, saturated fat, cholesterol and sodium, choose foods with a low % DV and don't go over 100% for the day. For total carbohydrate, dietary fiber, vitamins and minerals, your DV goal is to reach 100% of each.

Daily Values in the footnote are listed for people who eat 2,000 or 2,500 calories each day. If you eat more than 2,000 calories, your personal DV goals may exceed 100%. If you eat less, your personal DV goals will be lower.

Macaroni & Cheese

Nutrition Facts

Serving Size 1 cup (228g)
Servings Per Container 2

Amount Per Serving

Calories 250   Calories from Fat 110

	% Daily Value*
Total Fat 12g	18%
Saturated Fat 3g	15%
Cholesterol 30mg	10%
Sodium 470mg	20%
Total Carbohydrate 31g	10%
Dietary Fiber 0g	0%
Sugars 5g	
Protein 5g	

Vitamin A	4%	Vitamin C	2%
Calcium	20%	Iron	4%

* Percent Daily Values are based on a 2,000 calorie diet. Your daily values may be higher or lower depending on your calorie needs:

	Calories	2,000	2,500
Total Fat	Less than	65g	80g
Sat Fat	Less than	20g	25g
Cholesterol	Less than	300mg	300mg
Sodium	Less than	2,400mg	2,400mg
Total Carbohydrate		300g	375g
Dietary Fiber		25g	30g

Calories per gram:
Fat 9   •   Carbohydrate 4   •   Protein 4

Limit these nutrients.

Get enough of these nutrients.

5% or less is low. 20% or more is high.

More nutrients may be listed on some labels.

g = grams (About 28 g = 1 ounce)
mg = milligrams (1,000 mg = 1 g)

Serving Size

Is your serving the same size as the one on the label? If you eat double the serving size listed, you need to double the nutrient and calorie values. If you eat one-half the serving size shown here, cut the nutrient and calorie values in half.

Calories

Are you overweight? Cut back a little on calories! Look here to see how a serving of the food adds to your daily total. A 5' 4", 138-lb. active woman needs about 2,200 calories each day. A 5' 10", 174-lb. active man needs about 2,900. How about you? (Note: Fat-free is not calorie-free!)

Total Carbohydrate

When you cut down on fat, you can eat more carbohydrates. Carbohydrates are in foods like bread, potatoes, fruits and vegetables. Choose these often! They give you nutrients and energy.

Dietary Fiber

Grandmother called it "roughage," but her advice to eat more is still up-to-date! That goes for both soluble and insoluble kinds of dietary fiber. Fruits, vegetables, whole-grain foods, beans and peas are all good sources and can help reduce the risk of heart disease and cancer.

Protein

Most Americans get more protein than they need. Where there is animal protein, there is also fat and cholesterol. Eat small servings of lean meat, fish and poultry. Use fat-free or low-fat milk, yogurt and cheese. Try vegetable proteins like beans, grains and cereals.

Vitamins & Minerals

Your goal here is 100% of each for the day. Don't count on one food to do it all. Let a combination of foods add up to a winning score. New guidelines say teenagers need 1,300 mg of calcium per day (130% of Daily Value). Women after menopause need 1,500 mg of calcium (150% of Daily Value). 100% DV for calcium is 1,000 mg.

MAKE A PLAN

		Special Considerations
WHO		
WHERE		
WHEN		
HOW		
NEEDS		

MEDICATIONS
Things You Should Know

Every person should be able to answer the following questions before taking any new medication:

1. What is the name of the medication, and what is it supposed to do?

2. When and how do I take it?

3. How long should I take it?

4. Does this medication contain anything that can cause an allergic reaction?

5. Should I avoid alcohol, any other medicines, foods, and /or activities?

6. Should I expect any side effects?

7. What if I forget to take my medication?

8. Is it safe to become pregnant or to breast-feed while taking this medication

9. Is there a generic version of the medication that my physician has prescribed?

10. How should I store my medication?

Provided by Lisa Preimesberger, Pharm. D.
Adapted from American Pharmaceutical Association literature

Medications Quiz

		true	false
1.	My medicine is my doctor's responsibility. My job is just to take what the doctor gives me.	T	F
2.	The "medicine cabinet" in my bathroom is the best place to store my medicines.	T	F
3.	I should not stop taking my medicine, even if I begin to feel better before it's all gone.	T	F
4.	If I accidentally miss a dose, I should NOT take a double dose the next time.	T	F
5.	I need to call my doctor right away if I am having any serious side effects from the medication.	T	F
6.	My doctor's and pharmacist's instructions about how to take my medicine are just "guidelines."	T	F
7.	Never take medicine prescribed for someone else.	T	F

Answers:
1. False
2. False
3. True
4. True
5. True
6. False
7. True

Provided by Lisa Preimesberger, Pharm. D.
Adapted from American Pharmaceutical Association literature

PEOPLE — PLACES — EVENTS

PLACES - List 3 places you would enjoy visiting.

1. _____
2. _____
3. _____

EVENTS - List 3 events that you would like to do or take part in.

1. _____
2. _____
3. _____

PEOPLE - List 3 people with whom you would enjoy doing something.

1. _____
2. _____
3. _____

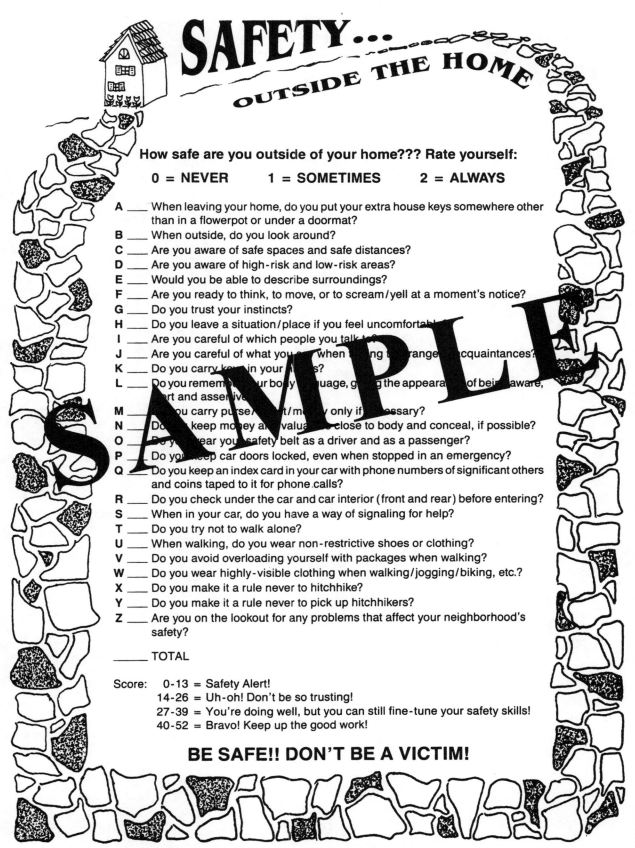

SAFETY...
OUTSIDE THE HOME

How safe are you outside of your home??? Rate yourself:

0 = NEVER   1 = SOMETIMES   2 = ALWAYS

A ____ When leaving your home, do you put your extra house keys somewhere other than in a flowerpot or under a doormat?

B ____ When outside, do you look around?

C ____ Are you aware of safe spaces and safe distances?

D ____ Are you aware of high-risk and low-risk areas?

E ____ Would you be able to describe surroundings?

F ____ Are you ready to think, to move, or to scream/yell at a moment's notice?

G ____ Do you trust your instincts?

H ____ Do you leave a situation/place if you feel uncomfortable?

I ____ Are you careful of which people you talk to?

J ____ Are you careful of what you say when talking to strangers/acquaintances?

K ____ Do you carry keys in your hands?

L ____ Do you remember your body language, giving the appearance of being aware, alert and assertive?

M ____ Do you carry purse/wallet/money only if necessary?

N ____ Do you keep money and valuables close to body and conceal, if possible?

O ____ Do you wear your safety belt as a driver and as a passenger?

P ____ Do you keep car doors locked, even when stopped in an emergency?

Q ____ Do you keep an index card in your car with phone numbers of significant others and coins taped to it for phone calls?

R ____ Do you check under the car and car interior (front and rear) before entering?

S ____ When in your car, do you have a way of signaling for help?

T ____ Do you try not to walk alone?

U ____ When walking, do you wear non-restrictive shoes or clothing?

V ____ Do you avoid overloading yourself with packages when walking?

W ____ Do you wear highly-visible clothing when walking/jogging/biking, etc.?

X ____ Do you make it a rule never to hitchhike?

Y ____ Do you make it a rule never to pick up hitchhikers?

Z ____ Are you on the lookout for any problems that affect your neighborhood's safety?

_____ TOTAL

Score: 0-13 = Safety Alert!
         14-26 = Uh-oh! Don't be so trusting!
         27-39 = You're doing well, but you can still fine-tune your safety skills!
         40-52 = Bravo! Keep up the good work!

BE SAFE!! DON'T BE A VICTIM!

Safety Tips to Prevent Falls

What are the causes of falls?

- Accident; environment related
- Muscle weakness
- Coordination or balance problem
- Dizziness, lightheadedness, vertigo
- Confusion
- Postural hypotension
- Impaired reflexes
- Vision or hearing impairment

Where do most falls occur?

- Bathroom and kitchen
- Areas with poor lighting
- Steps and stairs

How can you prevent falls?

- Identify potential risk factors early.
- Take your time; nothing is so important that you should risk falling.
- Use caution when getting up quickly or changing positions.
- Have your vision and hearing tested regularly and properly corrected if necessary.
- Talk to your doctor or pharmacist about the side effects of the medications you are taking and whether they affect your coordination or balance.

- Limit your intake of alcohol. Even a small amount of alcohol can disturb already impaired balance and reflexes.
- Make sure that the temperature in your home is at least 65° F during the night. Prolonged exposure to cold temperatures may cause a drop in body temperatures, which may lead to dizziness and falls.
- Use a cane or a walker to help maintain balance on uneven or unfamiliar ground and if you are prone to feeling dizzy. Use special caution in walking outdoors on wet and icy pavement.
- Wear supportive rubber-soled and low-heeled shoes. Avoid wearing smooth-soled slippers or socks on stairs and waxed floors. Floor surfaces should be clean, but not highly polished.
- Make your home safer with good lighting and minimal clutter. Have light switches installed at both the bottom and top of stairs.
- Use bedside light switches or night-lights.
- Be certain that both sides of stairways have sturdy handrails.
- Tack down carpeting on stairways and use nonskid treads.
- Use nonskid mats and throw rugs. Remove rugs if they tend to slide or curl up on the edges.
- Arrange furniture and other objects so as not to create an obstacle.
- Use grab bars on bathroom walls and nonskid mats or strips in the bathtub.
- In the living room, move electrical cords and telephone wires away from walkways.
- Make sure couches and chairs are at the proper height in order to stand up easily.
- Keep outdoor steps and walkways in good repair.
- Maintain a regular program of exercise in order to improve muscle strength and tone and to keep your joints more flexible. Check with your doctor or therapist to plan a suitable exercise program.

Sample Community Transportation Resources

Dial-a-Ride

(818) 405-4094	for application
(818) 398-0878	to schedule rides up to two weeks in advance

Area: Pasadena, San Marino, Altadena, LA County

Requirements: 60+ years old OR <60 with a disability

Cost: Free membership
$0.50/ride (may bring a guest for the same price)
Regular escorts ride free

Drawbacks: Must reserve pick-up ahead of time
Not direct, point to point service

Hints: For small groups, one person can arrange by giving everyone's name and card number

Access Services

1-800-827-0829	customer service
1-800-827-1359	hearing impaired

Area: LA County, San Gabriel Valley, Long Beach

Requirements: Must qualify for temporary or permanent disability

Cost: Free membership
$1.50/ride

Hints: Make ride appointment two hours before pick-up

Sample Group Feedback
How Does Transportation Affect Occupation?

Answers generated by group participants:

1. Transportation is necessary for many activities (such as shopping and visiting friends).

2. Transportation → Health → Activity
   For example, waiting for buses and transfers can make you late, tired, and stressed affecting your level of activity.

3. Transportation broadens awareness of the environment and may lead to more opportunities for occupation.

4. Transportation is a means to an end.

5. Transportation is also an occupation itself (for example, sightseeing).

6. Occupation is important for successful transportation. You must be able to obtain bus schedule information, travel times, directions, and so forth.

7. Transportation → Communication and interaction → Occupation

8. You can engage in occupation during transportation (for example, listening to the radio or reading).

Sample Group Feedback
How to Incorporate Exercise into Daily Life

1. Walk as much as possible for leisure or means of transportation.

2. Add extra movement to normal activities (for example, kick your legs while watching television).

3. Do your own cooking.

4. Use the stairs whenever possible.

5. Make exercise a routine.

6. Choose exercise that is fun.

7. Know that you can always take a break during exercise.

8. Exercise with friends (who do more moving than talking)!

Sample Summary of a
Nutrition and Medication Lecture

Things to do:
- Read labels on all medications
- Follow directions on label
- Be aware of side effects
- Inform your doctor of all medications you take
- Keep a list of medications for emergencies
- Update medicine cabinet once a year

Things NOT to do:
- Do not share medications with others
- Do not drink alcohol with medications (unless OK with doctor)
- Do not drive while taking certain medications
- Do not use a nasal decongestant if taking blood pressure medication

Medications can affect nutrition:

Medication	Foods to Avoid
Antibiotic	soda, citrus, and vegetable juice
Tetracycline	milk and dairy
Anti-coagulant	spinach, liver, and cabbage

Helpful hints:

- Cook with canola, olive, or peanut oil
- Add fiber to your diet gradually and with water
- When you drink caffeine, be sure to drink extra water
- Don't be fooled! Ground turkey has a lot of fat; aim for turkey breast
- Eat a variety of foods to ensure minimal exposure to toxic substances and increase your chances of receiving important nutrients
- Add fish to your diet to receive unique and healthy effects
- Use calcium citrate or carbonate
- Refer to the food guide pyramid to guide your daily food group amounts

Sample Summary of Police Safety Lecture

Always be <u>alert</u> and <u>aware</u> and <u>avoid</u> danger!

The biggest problem with street crime and the elderly is that seniors are usually injured during a crime. For example, a broken hip may result from being knocked down during a purse snatching.

- Keep distance between you and danger

- Think, plan, and dress for your outings (i.e. keep important items in a pocket, waist pack, or pinned under clothing)

- Be aware of scams and con-artists

- Don't display money in public

- Use direct deposit for Social Security payments

- Never give your credit card number over the phone unless you initiate the call

- Assert your rights

- Go to a crowded area and call attention to yourself in you need help

- No place is completely safe; always be prepared

- Report crime or suspicious activity immediately

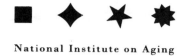

National Institute on Aging

What's Your Aging I.Q.?

	True	False
1. Baby boomers are the fastest growing segment of the population.	☐	☐
2. Families don't bother with their older relatives.	☐	☐
3. Everyone becomes confused or forgetful if they live long enough.	☐	☐
4. You can be too old to exercise.	☐	☐
5. Heart disease is a much bigger problem for older men than for older women.	☐	☐
6. The older you get, the less you sleep.	☐	☐
7. People should watch their weight as they age.	☐	☐
8. Most older people are depressed. Why shouldn't they be?	☐	☐
9. There's no point in screening older people for cancer because they can't be treated.	☐	☐
10. Older people take more medications than younger people.	☐	☐
11. People begin to lose interest in sex around age 55.	☐	☐
12. If your parents had Alzheimer's disease, you will inevitably get it.	☐	☐
13. Diet and exercise reduce the risk for osteoporosis.	☐	☐
14. As your body changes with age, so does your personality.	☐	☐
15. Older people might as well accept urinary accidents as a fact of life.	☐	☐
16. Suicide is mainly a problem for teenagers.	☐	☐
17. Falls and injuries "just happen" to older people.	☐	☐
18. Everybody gets cataracts.	☐	☐
19. Extremes of heat and cold can be especially dangerous for older people.	☐	☐
20. "You can't teach an old dog new tricks."	☐	☐

Answers

1. **False**.

There are more than 3 million Americans over the age of 85. That number is expected to quadruple by the year 2040, when there will be more than 12 million people in that age group. The population age 85 and older is the fastest growing age group in the U.S.

2 **False**.

Most older people live close to their children and see them often. Many live with their spouses. An estimated 80 percent of men and 60 percent of women live in family settings. Only 5 percent of the older population lives in nursing homes.

3. **False**.

Confusion and serious forgetfulness in old age can be caused by Alzheimer's disease or other conditions that result in irreversible damage to the brain. But at least 100 other problems can bring on the same symptoms. A minor head injury, high fever, poor nutrition, adverse drug reactions, and depression also can lead to confusion. These conditions are treatable, however, and the confusion they cause can be eliminated.

4. **False**.

Exercise at any age can help strengthen the heart and lungs and lower blood pressure. It also can improve muscle strength and, if carefully chosen, lessen bone loss with age. See a physician before beginning a new exercise program.

5. **False**.

The risk of heart disease increases dramatically for women after menopause. By age 65, both men and women have a one in three chance of showing symptoms. But risks can be significantly reduced by following a healthy diet and exercising.

6. **False**.

In later life, it's the quality of sleep that declines, not total sleep time. Researchers have found that sleep tends to become more fragmented as people age. A number of reports suggest that older people are less likely than younger people to stay awake throughout the day and that older people tend to take more naps than younger people.

7. **True**.

Most people gain weight as they age. Because of changes in the body and decreasing physical activity, older people usually need fewer calories. Still, a balanced diet is important. Older people require essential nutrients just like younger adults. You should be concerned about your weight if there has been an involuntary gain or loss of 10 pounds in the past 6 months.

8. **False**.

Most older people are not depressed. When it does occur, depression is treatable throughout the life cycle using a variety of approaches, such as family support, psychotherapy, or antidepressant medications. A physician can determine whether the depression is caused by medication an older person might be taking, by physical illness, stress, or other factors.

9. **False**.

Many older people can beat cancer, especially if it's found early. Over half of all cancers occur in people 65 and older, which means that screening for cancer in this age group is especially important.

10. **True**.

Older people often have a combination of conditions that require drugs. They consume 25 percent of all medications and can have many more problems with adverse reactions. Check with your doctor to make sure all drugs and dosages are appropriate.

11. False.

Most older people can lead an active, satisfying sex life.

12. False.

The overwhelming number of people with Alzheimer's disease have not inherited the disorder. In a few families, scientists have seen an extremely high incidence of the disease and have identified genes in these families which they think may be responsible.

13. True.

Women are at particular risk for osteoporosis. They can help prevent bone loss by eating foods rich in calcium and exercising regularly throughout life. Foods such as milk and other dairy products, dark green leafy vegetables, salmon, sardines, and tofu promote new bone growth. Activities such as walking, biking, and simple exercises to strengthen the upper body also can be effective.

14. False.

Research has found that, except for the changes that can result from Alzheimer's disease and other forms of dementia, personality is one of the few constants of life. That is, you are likely to age much as you've lived.

15. False.

Urinary incontinence is a symptom, not a disease. Usually, it is caused by specific changes in body function that can result from infection, diseases, pregnancy, or the use of certain medications. A variety of treatment options are available for people who seek medical attention.

16. False.

Suicide is most prevalent among people age 65 and older. An older person's concern with suicide should be taken very seriously and professional help should be sought quickly.

17. False.

Falls are the most common cause of injuries among people over age 65. But many of these injuries, which result in broken bones, can be avoided. Regular vision and hearing tests and good safety habits can help prevent accidents. Knowing whether your medications affect balance and coordination also is a good idea.

18. False.

Not everyone gets cataracts, although a great many older people do. Some 18 percent of people between the ages of 65 and 74 have cataracts, while more than 40 percent of those between 75 and 85 have the problem. Cataracts can be treated very successfully with surgery; more than 90 percent of people say they can see better after the procedure.

19. True.

The body's thermostat tends to function less efficiently with age, making the older person's body less able to adapt to heat or cold.

20. False.

People at any age can learn new information and skills. Research indicates that older people can obtain new skills and improve old ones, including how to use a computer.

U.S. DEPARTMENT OF HEALTH AND HUMAN SERVICES
Public Health Service
National Institutes of Health
October 1991
U.S. Government Printing Office: 1991—281–837/40019

Words of Wisdom from Healthy Seniors:
What Does it Mean to be Healthy?

Below are 25 ways to be healthy…

1. Maintain proper diet and nutrition
2. Engage in physical exercise
3. Schedule regular physical check-ups
4. Drink plenty of water
5. Take proper medication and use correct equipment
6. Involve your mind in mental exercise (i.e. games, puzzles)
7. Take time for rest and relaxation
8. Find recreational occupations
9. Try new and amusing activities
10. Participate in enjoyable occupations (i.e. music, cultural events, bingo)
11. Have a balance of activities
12. Meditate
13. Nurture your spiritual life
14. Take tea or coffee breaks
15. Keep a positive mindset – an "I can do" attitude
16. Visit and meet new people
17. Go to social events with friends
18. Create love and support in your life
19. Have a pet
20. Smile
21. Try a change of environment
22. Volunteer, provide service, and share knowledge
23. Live moderately; don't work too hard
24. Avoid trouble and worry
25. Learn to be happy

Appendix 4
Resource List

Audiovisual Materials

Arthritis and everyday living [Videotape]. (1987). (Available from A/V Health Services, Inc., P.O. Box 20271, Roanoke, VA 24018)

Harlowe, D. (Writer), & Yu, P. (Writer, Music, & Narrator). (1993a). *ROM relaxation: Body awareness & breathing* [Cassette Recording] . Madison, WI: St. Mary's Hospital Medical Center.

Harlowe, D. (Verse), & Yu, P. (Verse, Music, & Narration). (1993b). *The ROM dance: Seated version* [Cassette Recording]. Madison, WI: St. Mary's Hospital Medical Center.

Living younger longer: Real people getting real results [Videotape]. (1993). (Available from Living Younger Longer, Inc., P.O. Box 480124, Denver, CO 80248)

The sixth sense [Videotape]. (1985). (Available from The National Council on Aging, Inc., 409 Third Street SW, Washington, DC 20024)

Print Materials

Johnson, J. S. (1987). *Celebrating the familiar: The sculptures of J. Seward Johnson Jr*. New York: Alfred Van der Marck Editors.

Korb, K. L., Azok, S. D., & Leutenberg, E. A. (1991). *Life management skills II: Reproducible activity handouts created for facilitators*. Beachwood, OH: Wellness Reproductions.

Salmen, J. P. S. (1991). *The do-able renewable home: Making your home fit your needs*. Washington, DC: American Association of Retired Persons.

Organizations

American Academy of Family Physicians
8880 Ward Parkway
Kansas City, MO 64114
Telephone: (816) 333-9700
Internet address: www.aafp.org

American Dietetic Association
Telephone: (202) 371-0500
Internet address: www.eatright.org

American Heart Association
National Center
7272 Greenville Avenue
Dallas, TX 75231-4596
Telephone (Publications): (800) 787-8984

National Council on the Aging, Inc.
409 Third Street SW
Washington, DC 20024
Telephone: (202) 479-1200, (800) 424-9046
Internet address: www.ncoa.org

National Institute on Aging
(Age Pages and What's Your Aging I.Q.?)
NIA Information Center
P.O. Box 8057
Gaithersburg, MD 20898-8057
Telephone (Public Information Office): (301) 496-1752
Telephone (Publications): (800) 222-2225
TDD: (800) 222-4225

Nutrition Screening Initiative
(Determine Your Nutritional Health Checklist)
1010 Wisconsin Avenue NW
Suite 800

Washington, DC 20007
Telephone: (202) 625-1662

U.S. Food and Drug Administration
(Can Your Kitchen Pass the Food Safety Test?)
5600 Fishers Lane
Rockville, MD 20857
Telephone: (888) 322-4636
Internet address: www.fda.gov/comments.html

Wellness Reproductions, Inc.
(Life Management Skills activity handouts)
23945 Mercantile Road
Beachwood, OH 44122-5924
Telephone: (800) 669-9208

References

Addams, J. (1990). *Twenty years at Hull-House.* Chicago, IL: University of Illinois.

American Heritage Dictionary (2nd collegiate ed.). (1989). New York: Bantam.

Applegate, J. S., & Bonovitz, J. M. (1995). *The facilitating partnership: A Winnicottian approach for social workers and other helping professionals.* Northvale, NJ: Aronson.

Belenky, M. F., Bond, L. A., & Weinstock, J. S. (1997). A tradition that has no name: Nurturing the development of people, families, and communities. New York: Basic Books.

Bender, M., Norris, A., & Bauckham, P. (1991). Groupwork with the elderly: Principles and practice. Oxon, United Kingdom: Winslow Press.

Bergner, M., Bobbitt, R. A., Carter, W. B., & Gilson, B. S. (1981). The sickness impact profile: Validation of a health status measure. *Med Care, 14,* 57–70.

Billings, J. R., & Cowley, S. C. (1995). Approaches to community needs assessment: A literature review. *Journal of Advanced Nursing, 22,* 721–730.

Borg, B., & Bruce, M. G. (1991). *The group system: The therapeutic activity group in occupational therapy.* Thorofare, NJ: Slack.

Brown, R. (1988). *Group processes: Dynamics within and between groups.* Oxford, England: Basil Blackwell.

Bruce, M., & Borg, B. (1993). *Psychosocial occupational therapy: Frames of reference for intervention* (2nd ed.). Thorofare, NJ: Slack.

Burke, J. P., & Cassidy, J. C. (1991). Disparity between reimbursement-driven practice and humanistic values of occupational therapy. *American Journal of Occupational Therapy, 45,* 173–176.

Burnside, I. M. (1978). *Working with the elderly: Group process and techniques.* North Scituate, MA: Duxbury.

Carlson, M., Clark, F., & Young, B. (1998). Practical contributions of occupational science to the art of successful aging: How to sculpt a meaningful life in older adulthood. *Journal of Occupational Science, 5,* 107–118.

Carlson, M., Fanchiang, S., Zemke, R., & Clark, F. (1996). A meta-analysis of the effectiveness of occupational therapy for older persons. *American Journal of Occupational Therapy, 50,* 89–98.

Clark, F. (1997). Reflections on the human as an occupational being: Biological need, tempo and temporality. *Journal of Occupational Science Australia, 4,* 86–92.

Clark, F. A. (1993). Occupation embedded in a real life: Interweaving occupational science and occupational therapy. 1993 Eleanor Clarke Slagle lecture. *American Journal of Occupational Therapy, 47,* 1067–1078.

Clark, F., Azen, S., Carlson, M., Mandel, D., Zemke, R., Hay, J., Luo, R., & LaBree, L. (1999). *Occupational therapy for independent-living older adults: Long-term follow-up.* Manuscript submitted for publication.

Clark, F., Azen, S., Zemke, R., Jackson, J., Carlson, M., Mandel, D., Hay, J., Josephson, K., Cherry, B., Hessel, C., Palmer, J., & Lipson, L. (1997). Occupational therapy for independent-living older adults: A randomized controlled trial. *Journal of the American Medical Association, 278,* 1321–1326.

Clark, F., Carlson, M., Zemke, R., Frank, G., Patterson, K., Ennevor, B. L., Rankin-Martinez, A., Hobson, L., Crandall, J., Mandel, D., & Lipson, L. (1996). Life domains and adaptive strategies of a group of low-income well older adults. *American Journal of Occupational Therapy, 50,* 99–108.

Clark, F., Ennevor, B. L., & Richardson, P. L. (1996). A grounded theory of techniques for occupational storytelling and occupational story making. In R. Zemke & F. Clark (Eds.), *Occupational science: The evolving discipline* (pp. 373–392). Philadelphia: F. A. Davis.

Clark, F., Parham, D., Carlson, M. E., Frank, G., Jackson, J., Peirce, D., Wolfe, R. J., & Zemke, R. (1991). Occupational science: Academic innovation in the service of occupational therapy's future. *American Journal of Occupational Therapy, 45,* 300–310.

Clark, F., Wood, W., & Larson, E. A. (1998). Occupational science: Occupational therapy's legacy for the 21st century. In M. E. Neistadt & E. B. Crepeau (Eds.), *Willard & Spackman's occupational therapy* (pp. 13–21). Philadelphia: Lippincott-Raven.

Cole, M. B. (1998). *Group dynamics in occupational therapy: The theoretical basis and practice application of group treatment* (2nd ed.). Thorofare, NJ: Slack.

Coyne, J. C., & Calarco, M. M. (1995). Effects of the experience of depression: Application of focus group and survey methodologies. *Psychiatry, 58,* 149–163.

Crimmins, E. M., Hayward, M. D., & Saito, Y. (1994). Changing mortality and morbidity rates and the health status and life expectancy of the older population. *Demography, 31,* 159–175.

Csikszentmihalyi, M. (1990). *Flow: The psychology of optimal experience.* New York: Harper & Row.

Dunton, W. R. (1915). *Occupation therapy: A manual for nurses.* Philadelphia: Saunders.

Englehardt, H. T. (1977). Defining occupational therapy: The meaning of therapy and the virtues of occupation. *American Journal of Occupational Therapy, 31*, 666–672.

Fazio, L. S. (1992). Tell me a story: The therapeutic metaphor in the practice of pediatric occupational therapy. *American Journal of Occupational Therapy, 46*, 112–119.

Forer, S. (1996). *Outcome management and program evaluation made easy: A toolkit for occupational therapy practitioners.* Bethesda, MD: American Occupational Therapy Association.

Frankl, V. (1969). *The will to meaning.* New York: World Publishing.

Giddens, A. (1991). *Modernity and self-identity: Self and society in late modern age.* Stanford, CA: Stanford University Press.

Hall, H. J. (1918). Arts and crafts in medicine. *Proceedings of the 1st annual meeting of the National Society for the Promotion of Occupational Therapy* (pp. 38–41). Towson, MD: National Society for the Promotion of Occupational Therapy.

Hays, R. D., Sherbourne, C. D., & Mazel, R. M. (1993). The RAND 36-Item Health Survey 1.0. *Health Economy, 2*, 217–227.

Hays, V., Morris, J., Wolfe, C., & Morgan, M. (1995). The SF-36 Health Survey Questionnaire: Is it suitable for use with older adults? *Age and Aging, 24*, 120–125.

Howe, M. C., & Schwartzberg, S. L. (1995). *A functional approach to group work in occupational therapy* (2nd ed.). Philadelphia: Lippincott.

Jackson, J. (1996). Living a meaningful existence in old age. In R. Zemke & F. Clark (Eds.), *Occupational science: The evolving discipline* (pp. 339–361). Philadelphia: F. A. Davis.

Jackson, J., Carlson, M., Mandel, D., Zemke, R., & Clark, F. (1998). Occupation in lifestyle redesign: The well elderly study occupational therapy program. *American Journal of Occupational Therapy, 52*, 326–336.

Jette, A. M., & Cleary, P. D. (1987). Functional disability assessment. *Physical Therapy, 67*, 1854–1859.

Johnson, J. (1986). *Wellness: A context for living.* Thorofare, NJ: Slack.

Kaufman, S. R. (1986). *The ageless self: Sources of meaning in late life.* Madison, WI: University of Wisconsin Press.

Kniepmann, K. (1997). Prevention of disability and maintenance of health. In C. H. Christiansen & C. M. Baum (Eds.), *Occupational therapy: Enabling function and well-being* (pp. 530–555). Thorofare, NJ: Slack.

Krupnick, W. (1996). The targeting of communications. In M. Johnson (Ed.), *The occupational therapy manager* (pp. 117–141). Bethesda, MD: American Occupational Therapy Association.

Lautar, C. (1996). A focus group study: Overview of the methodology. *Probe, 30*, 53–56.

Lave, J., & Wenger, E. (1991). *Situated learning: Legitimate peripheral participation.* Cambridge, United Kingdom: Cambridge University.

Law, M., Baptiste, S., McColl, M. A., Carswell, A., Polatajko, H., & Pollock, N. (1994). *Canadian Occupational Performance Measure* (2nd ed.). Toronto, Ontario, Canada: Canadian Association of Occupational Therapists.

Lincoln, Y. S., & Guba, E. G. (1981). *Effective evaluation.* San Francisco: Jossey-Bass.

Malec, J. F., Smigielski, J. S., & DePompolo, R. W. (1991). Goal attainment scaling and outcome measurement in postacute brain injury rehabilitation. *Archives of Physical Medicine and Rehabilitation, 72*, 138–143.

Mandel, D. (Producer), & Roy, B. (Director). (1995). *I CAN* [Film]. (Available from USC Department of Occupational Science and Occupational Therapy, 1540 Alcazar Street, CHP-133, Los Angeles, CA, 90033)

Mangione, C. M., Goldman, L., Orav, E. J., Marcantonio, E. R., Pedan, A., Ludwig, L. E., Donaldson, M. C., Sugarbaker, D. J., Poss, R., & Lee, T. H. (1997). Health-related quality of life after elective surgery: Measurement of longitudinal changes. *Journal of General Internal Medicine, 12*, 686–697.

Manning, D. (1984). *Don't take my grief away: What to do when you lose a loved one.* San Francisco: Harper.

Maslow, A. H. (1987). *Motivation and personality* (3rd ed.). New York: Harper & Row.

McHorney, C. A., Ware, J. E., & Raczek, A. E. (1993). The MOS 36-Item Short Form Health Survey (SF-36): II. Psychometric and clinical tests of validity in measuring physical and mental health constructs. *Medical Care, 31*, 247–263.

Meyer, A. (1977). The philosophy of occupation therapy. *American Journal of Occupational Therapy, 31*, 639–642.

Millar, B., Maggs, C., Warner, V., & Whale, Z. (1996). Creating consensus about nursing outcomes. I: An exploration of focus group methodology. *Journal of Clinical Nursing, 5*, 193–197.

Morgan, D. L. (1997). *Focus groups as qualitative research* (2nd ed.). London: Sage.

Ornstein, R., & Sobel, D. (1989). *Healthy pleasures.* Reading, MA: Addison-Wesley.

Ory, M. G., & Cox, D. M. (1994). Forging ahead: Linking health and behavior to improve quality of life in older people. *Social Indicators Research, 33*, 89–120.

Ottenbacher, K. J., & Cusick, A. (1990). Goal attainment scaling as a method of clinical service evaluation. *American Journal of Occupational Therapy, 44*, 519–525.

Peloquin, S. M. (1991a). Occupational therapy service: Individual and collective understandings of the founders: Part 1. *American Journal of Occupational Therapy, 45*, 352–360.

Peloquin, S. M. (1991b). Occupational therapy service: Individual and collective understandings of the founders: Part 2. *American Journal of Occupational Therapy, 45*, 733–744.

Polit, D. F., & Hungler, B. P. (1991). *Nursing research: Principles and methods*. Philadelphia: Lippincott.

Price-Lackey, P., & Cashman, J. (1996). Jenny's story: Reinventing oneself through occupation and narrative configuration. *American Journal of Occupational Therapy, 50*, 306–314.

Radloff, L. (1977). The CES-D Scale: A self-report depression scale for research in the general population. *Applied Psychological Measures, 1*, 385–401.

Reed, K. L. (1986). Tools of practice: Heritage or baggage? *American Journal of Occupational Therapy, 40*, 597–605.

Reich, J. W., & Zautra, A. J. (1991). Analyzing the trait of routinization in older adults. *International Journal of Aging and Human Development, 32*, 161–180.

Roberts, K. B. (1996). Educational principles of community-based education. *Pediatrics, 98*, 1259–1263.

Rogers, C. R. (1980). *A way of being*. Boston: Houghton Mifflin.

Rowe, J. W., & Kahn, R. L. (1998). *Successful aging*. New York: Pantheon Books.

Schwartzberg, S. L. (1998). Group process. In M. E. Neistadt & E. B. Crepeau (Eds.), *Willard & Spackman's occupational therapy* (pp. 120–131). Philadelphia: Lippincott.

Slagle, E. C. (1921, October). *Training aides for mental patients*. Paper presented at the 5th annual meeting of the National Society for the Promotion of Occupational Therapy, Baltimore, MD.

Stewart, A. L., Hays, R. D., & Ware, J. E. (1988). The MOS Short-Form General Health Survey. *Medical Care, 26*, 724–735.

Stewart, D. W., & Shamdasani, P. N. (1990). *Focus groups: Theory and practice*. London: Sage.

Tarlov, A. R., Ware, J. E., Greenfield, S., Nelson, E. C., Perrin, E., & Zubkoff, M. (1989). The medical outcomes study: An application of methods for monitoring the results of medical care. *Journal of the American Medical Association, 26*, 925–930.

Templeton, J. F. (1987). *Focus groups: A guide for marketing & advertising professionals*. Chicago: Probus.

Toseland, R. W. (1995). *Group work with the elderly and family caregivers*. New York: Springer.

Tracy, S. E. (1912). *Studies in invalid occupation*. Boston: Whitcomb & Barrows.

Trombly, C. A., Vining, M., & Radomski, E. S. D. (1998). Achievement of self-identified goals by adults with traumatic brain injury: Phase I. *American Journal of Occupational Therapy, 52*, 810–818.

U.S. Bureau of the Census. (1992). *Current population reports: Special studies: Sixty-five plus in America* (Publication No. P23-178). Washington, DC: U.S. Government Printing Office.

U.S. Bureau of the Census (1996). *Statistical abstract of the US*. Washington, DC: U.S. Government Printing Office.

Ware, J. E., Kosinski, M., & Keller, S. K. (1994). *SF-36 Physical and Mental Health Summary Scales: A user's manual*. Boston: The Health Institute, New England Medical Center.

Ware, J. E., & Sherbourne, C. D. (1992). The MOS 36-Item Short-Form Health Survey (SF-36): I. *Medical Care, 30*, 473–481.

West, W. L. (1969). The growing importance of prevention. *American Journal of Occupational Therapy, 23*, 226–231.

West, W. L. (1990). Nationally Speaking—Perspectives on the past and future: Part 2. *American Journal of Occupational Therapy, 44*, 9–10.

Wood, V., Wylie, M. L., & Sheafor, B. (1969). An analysis of a short self-reported measure of life satisfaction. *Journal of Gerontology, 24*, 465–469.

Yerxa, E. J., Clark, F., Frank, G., Jackson, J., Parham, D., Pierce, D., Stein, C., & Zemke, R. (1989). An introduction to occupational science: A foundation for occupational therapy in the 21st century. *Occupational Therapy in Health Care, 6*, 1–17.